DEMENTIA CARERS' HANDBOOK

Practical Care and Coping Strategies for Service Users, Carers and Families

Emerson J. Jones

Shield Crest

ISBN: 978-1-912505-59-3

MMXIX

A CIP catalogue record for this book
is available from the British Library

Published by
ShieldCrest Publishing Ltd.,
Aylesbury, Buckinghamshire,
HP18 0TF England
Tel: +44 (0) 333 8000 890
www.shieldcrest.co.uk

Acknowledgements

There is explicit gratitude to fellow members of the Dementia Information and Support for Carers Organisation (DISC) whose views, shared experiences and insights I have drawn upon to develop, challenge and advance my own thinking in writing this handbook. This has enabled me to reinforce my understanding and to develop various coping strategies, key principles, best 'care' practices and tools for use by those caring for people with dementia.

To Valarie Morgan-Richards, DISC former deputy manager and dementia adviser, I owe an immense debt of gratitude for allowing me to draw on her experience and the offer of constructive comments in helping to make the contents relevant and for making this handbook possible.

Special thanks are due to Mandie Baker, DISC co-ordinator, South Birmingham, for her key contributions and advice on the many drafts submitted. Her inputs contained on several pages greatly contributed to the quality of this handbook.

To my fellow carer Dionne Saddler, many thanks for reviewing several chapters of the handbook and for giving generously her time and suggestions. Her comments and insights are invaluable and much appreciated.

Finally, to my daughters Jennifer and Sonia for their guidance at all stages of writing this book and who continuously gave me company during the journey. I am grateful to them both for helping to ensure a sustainable high standard of presentation was achieved and the many helpful suggestions for improving the usefulness of the handbook.

About the Author

Emerson J Jones is a carer with several years' experience in delivering home care and support for his wife with vascular dementia and Alzheimer's. This has enabled him to gain unique insights into the challenges and issues facing carers and families in the planning and delivery of appropriate and responsive quality care, as well as the impacts on carers' roles, responsibilities, health and wellbeing and lifestyle.

As a carer and inspired by the desire to contribute to the care and support for people with dementia, it has led him to develop approaches that would enable carers and families to better cope with their caring and supporting roles. Being a member of the Dementia Information and Support for Carers Organisation (DISC) he has written several articles on dementia care for the DISC Carers Newsletter.

Emerson has worked extensively with health and social care professionals and practitioners on the design of dementia care, support and services and on carer's needs and priorities. He has provided several written submissions on Dementia Strategy Framework, Dementia Carers Strategy, review of Community Day Care for Adults and the Carers Grant Scheme.

Emerson also served as a Member of the Scrutiny and Review Committee on Health and Social Care.

Contents

Introduction

A Dementia Care, Support and Resource Model for Caring Situations

The purpose of this handbook is to introduce strategies and plans for service users, carers and families supporting and caring for individuals living with dementia or Alzheimer's. It provides essential best practices for coping with the delivery of care during all stages of the dementia pathway.

It is designed with strategies for dealing with various behavioural challenges, cognitive impairments and functional disabilities that occur as the condition progresses.

The handbook also provides practical tools and templates that are needed for the delivery of compassionate, sustainable and responsive quality care, with a focus on developing the resilience of carers. It further aims to enhance the quality of life of people with dementia, improve the health and wellbeing of carers and families, the experience of carers and to achieve improved outcomes for all.

Finally the handbook is intended as a guide and resource for professionals and practitioners in health and social care disciplines. It aims to improve awareness and identification of carers issues so that they feel confident, supported and being heard when the person they care for is in a health and social care setting. However, it is not to be regarded as an exhaustive text, nor meant to be used as a standard of health or social care practice or as a substitute for professional and medical advice, but as an essential carers guide for dementia care and support – in this regard it can best be described as going on a journey with carers and ensuring carers formal support in their caring role.

Preface

Regarded as a global epidemic of the 21st Century, dementia is a complex illness that can have a devastating impact on the lives of people with the condition, their spouse or partner, families and friends, with challenges and changes in behaviour, communications and relationships.

Increasing life expectancy and the rise in age-related physical or mental disabilities are regarded as predisposing factors behind the rise in dementia. Other potential risk factors include: gender (Alzheimer's being slightly more common in females, vascular dementia more in males), head injury, genetics, lifestyle factors (diet, exercise, smoking and alcohol), medical conditions, such as diabetes, high blood pressure, high cholesterol, heart disease and history of stroke. Dementia is also considered as a natural reaction to the environment we live in.

In the United Kingdom it is estimated that there are over 850,000 people living with Alzheimer's or different types of dementias, with informal family carers or close friends providing homecare and support. This number is set to rise to over one million by 2025. While there is an increasing level of awareness of dementia in communities and that various levels of supportive social and healthcare services are in place, there is reliance upon informal family carers as the cornerstone of homecare and support. The impact on those receiving care at home by family members cannot always be measured, but may be regarded as profound and priceless.

Caring for a person with dementia is often an intensive, challenging, impactful and at times stressful experience. It places much greater demands and strains on family carers who are often challenged by emotional distress and physical exhaustion, with increasing levels of stress from coping with disturbing or uncontrollable situations or experiences. These are mainly regarded as common symptoms of 'compassion fatigue' or burnout. Caregiving demands also make it difficult for carers to cope with their own feelings – a situation that negatively impacts the quality of life for persons with dementia and those around them.

As the condition progresses, people living with dementia are often found having the highest level of social and healthcare needs, including quality care, support and services. Meanwhile carers and family members are faced with unique and extreme challenges of coping with changes in motivation, mood, memory, capability and behaviour that occur along various stages of the dementia pathway.

Dealing effectively with the symptoms of dementia will require an effective, coordinated and responsive health and social care programme. This is intended to delay the process of deterioration of the condition, prevent crisis situations in advanced stage of dementia, enhance carers' resilience and coping skills, and maintain carers' health and wellbeing.

This handbook introduces various interventions that combine different elements of support and services with a mix of responses, actions and practices. These are aimed at building the resilience of carers and families, improving the health and wellbeing of those involved, and safeguarding and upholding the dignity and self-respect of those cared for, geared towards enhancing the quality of life and achieving the desired outcomes for all.

About the Dementia Carers Handbook

Written for carers by carers, the Dementia Carers Handbook on Practical Care and Coping Strategies is for carers and families caring and supporting people living with various types of dementias and Alzheimer's disease. It is designed for easy reading, and selective and practical application of best practices for delivering compassionate and sustainable homecare.

The handbook is intended as a practical guide that allows carers and families to manage and better cope with the challenges of caring for those with the condition. It introduces strategies, approaches and best 'care' practices for coping with changes in behaviour and, in particular, dealing with non-compliant, resistive, aggressive, threatening and other types of challenging behaviours. Practice guidelines for health and social care professionals, support workers and service providers working with carers and families are included.

Many of the strategies have been developed drawing from a mix of knowledge and experience of people with dementia, professional and partner organisations, carers and families' reflections and insights in their home support and caring roles, conceptual discussions and document reviews and analysis of carers' support and needs. Various interventions and best practices in selected countries have been explored in depth, seeking available evidence of how best to understand and support carers and families caring for those with dementia.

The strategies outlined deal with topics that include lifestyle risk factors, carers' emotional health and wellbeing, safeguarding priorities, ensuring dignity, self-respect and quality of life, issues impacting carers' roles and ensuring balance in carers' lives and responsibilities. Key issues and findings relating to those with dementia, their carers and families from ethnic minority communities in providing culturally appropriate care, support and services are also analysed and discussed.

It is a handbook which provides benefits such as information and awareness of the support and service needs of carers, steps that minimise disruption to daily care and support routines, defines clear expectations of acceptable care practices, promotes better planning outcomes from caring, strengthens integrated and person-centred support and care, and improvements of the physical, emotional wellbeing and wellness of carers.

Finally the handbook is dedicated to all carers, families and friends facing significant challenges in providing the daily care and support needs of individuals. It involves coming to terms with varying levels of cognitive deficits with diminished or lack of functional capacity mostly among frail and elderly people with higher prevalence of chronic diseases and associated disabilities and dependencies. Various forms of behavioural manifestations faced by carers and families are also addressed.

The handbook is intended as a resource to promote independence, and for building the resilience of carers and families that will enable them to undertake their caring role in an intense, rewarding and fulfilling way, while aiming to enhance the quality and fulfilment of their lives.

A PATHWAY TO DEMENTIA CARE, SUPPORT AND SERVICES

Empowering People with Dementia, their Carers and Families through Information, Advice, Advocacy, Training, Support and Services delivered through multiple channels of intervention

Supporting Carers and Families in Managing and Coping With Alzheimer's and Dementia Care

SECTION I

Creating Awareness and Understanding of Dementia Care

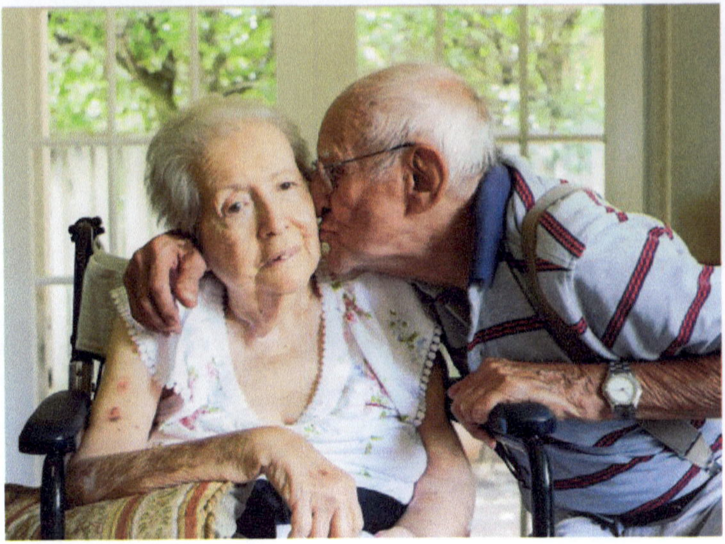

CHAPTER 1

Creating Awareness and Understanding of Dementia

Carers and families of persons living with dementia often face difficult challenges when providing the daily care and support needs for these individuals. Coping with changes in behaviour and the unpredictability of changes that occur throughout various stages of the dementia can be stressful, frustrating and physically and emotionally demanding for carers and families alike. As the dementia progresses, the individual may display many behavioural and personality traits in ways that are considered culturally inappropriate, threatening and aggressive, non-compliant and difficult to manage.

Behavioural symptoms can occur during various stages of dementia and may include repetitive questioning, agitation or restlessness, wandering, hoarding, sundowning and verbal or physical aggression. Psychological symptoms are also common features of people with dementia and usually involve anxiety, depressive moods, confusion, hallucinations and delusions.

The condition of dementia impacts on the person's memory, language, ability to communicate, mood and personality. These and other characteristics on which normal social, occupational and domestic life depends often become impaired. People with dementia may not experience all these symptoms; the degree to which they are experienced will also differ between individuals.

For carers it is often a life characterised by profound emotional and physical apathy that results from the constant demands of caring. This may eventually diminish the ability to feel empathy and compassion for those they care for, thus defeating the purpose of their role.

Cases of dementia are normally progressive in nature and are diagnosed as mild cognitive impairment/early stage dementia, mid-stage/moderate stage dementia, severe or advanced stage, and last or end of life stage, with clear and noticeable symptoms that occur at each stage.

For every stage of dementia a person may exhibit mild, moderate or severe behavioural and personality changes and manifestations, diminished or lack of capacity, functional and physical disabilities, including ability to perform or complete simple or complex tasks, gaps in memory or severe memory loss and impairment in visuo-spatial abilities.

As the dementia condition progresses the prevalence of symptoms and level of disability increases, resulting in heightened levels of risks to physical health. This is very much evident in advanced or last stage dementia, with frequently occurring symptoms such as pain and rigidity of the muscles, urinary and bowel incontinence, eating problems and loss of appetite, shortness of breath and lack of mobility, which all contribute to the need for greater care and appropriate support. This also underlines the need for health and social care practitioners to work collaboratively with family carers in the planning and delivery of care.

In developing the care plans for persons with dementia, and in cases where there is progression of the disease, carers and families should be made aware that dementia affects every person differently. Care options that work for one person may need to be adapted or changed in the future; a situation in which there will be need for constant adjustments to the caring situation, and for care and support to be adjusted to cope with conditions of behavioural disturbances, diminished capacity, memory loss and changes in abilities.

CHAPTER 2

Caring and Supporting People with Dementia: Issues and Challenges

The condition of dementia affects people across all ages, ethnicities and communities. It does not discriminate between professional or social status. Every person with dementia is different and how the illness affects an individual depends on which area of the brain is affected

Whatever form of dementia is diagnosed, and where there are symptoms of progression, the care, support and service needs of the person increases, as does the support needs of carers and families. Carers of people with dementia are regarded as critical to sustaining the quality of life, and for safeguarding and preserving the respect and dignity of the individual. It is also acknowledged that the health and emotional wellbeing of family carers relies heavily on the quality of support and services that are available and accessible in a timely way.

There are many factors to be considered that can influence the dementia homecare situation. From the onset of dementia, carers and families are frequently faced with a lack of understanding of the condition, their role as carers, and the system of care, support and services available often appear complex and fragmented. This makes it difficult to navigate and coordinate many aspects of the care and support system on their own.

Where multiple agencies are involved in a person's care, advice, support and service needs are often difficult to access and confusing for families to use. Carers may also lack specific dementia care skills and knowledge, coupled with the difficulty in gaining referrals and access to information. Service providers are often viewed as lacking understanding, care and compassion, and being inflexible and reactive at times. Carers often feel there is a lack of quality in the choice of services they need, particularly for respite or day care.

For people with dementia and associated disabilities, they are at a greater risk than others, such as older people and minorities. Many of these individuals run the risk of becoming disadvantaged in society and not understanding their rights due to illness, age or culture.

Carers should always endeavour to advance and protect their rights to independence, self-fulfilment, self-care, good healthcare, and participate in their community.

These are considerations that have implications for: awareness and understanding issues of dignity; change in public perception of dementia; education and training needs of carers and family members; considering and facilitating the cultural and linguistic requirements of each individual, and safeguarding the rights of those at risk.

As the care and support needs increase, and in trying to adapt or cope with the obvious difficulties that often occur, carers may often experience feelings of frustration, irritability, guilt, anger, loneliness and social isolation as a result of physical and emotional fatigue and apathy. This is sometimes accompanied with intense feelings that their needs are not being met or understood. Also common are the difficulties of emotional acceptance of their caring role and adjusting to caring and supporting realities.

These are feelings, that if remain unaddressed, may lead to anxiety and depression, with increased risk of significant health problems. Such conditions could eventually affect the carers' wellbeing and quality of life of those cared for.

SECTION II

Identifying and Accessing Coping Strategies

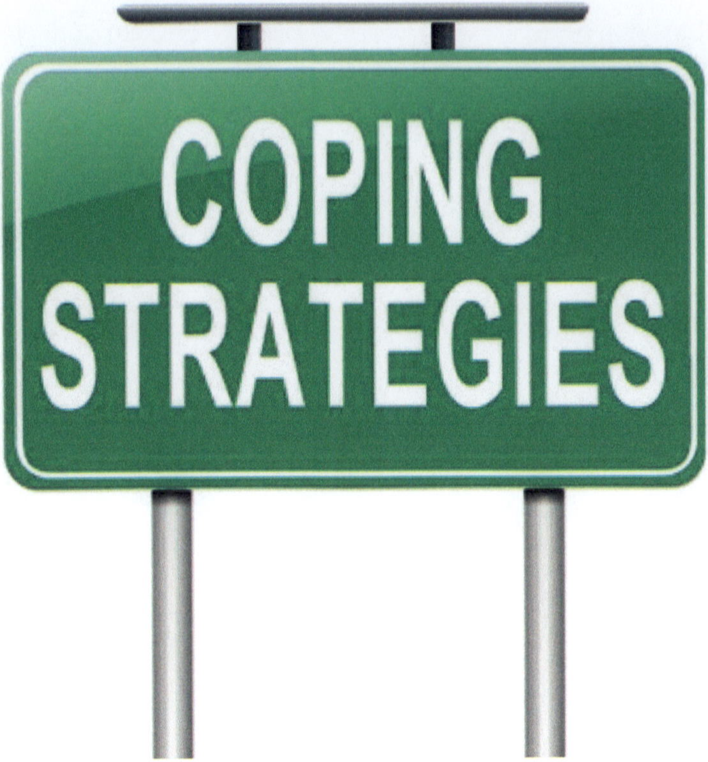

CHAPTER 3

Use of Coping Strategies for Carers and Families

In managing the daily care needs of a person with dementia, carers may often become overwhelmed with the burdens and demands of caring and are susceptible to stresses that affect their physical, mental and emotional health and wellbeing.

The knowledge and use of coping strategies could provide carers with insights, and the ability to adapt and adjust to changes and experiences in their caring routines and tasks.

Coping strategies involve a mix of responses, actions and practices that enable carers to deal with the daily pressures of caring, and can be used for coping with different kinds of dementia challenged behaviours. The use of coping strategies will also enable carers to remain engaged and active whilst retaining a sense of control over their daily lives.

Carers and families may also find coping strategies as a way of finding solutions for many care-related issues and challenges, targeting specific or common forms of behaviours.

The use of coping strategies is subjective and may be triggered by or as a response to various conditions associated with the carer's personal experience, such as the carer and/or the person's environment, type of communication, nature of the tasks the carer may attempt to undertake, and a health condition which the person may be unable to understand or communicate.

Dementia coping strategies can be used in the following ways:

- Changes and challenges in the behaviour of persons, including the frequency of different types of behaviours and how these affect the carers' role and duties.
- The person's progressive lack of ability or significantly diminished physical, mental and functional capacity to perform daily or simple activities or tasks.
- In support of effective care management and delivery processes.
- The struggle to balance carers' responsibilities with working life.
- As a tool used for carers' support and the delivery of dementia care.
- As a resource for health and social care professionals.
- Provides the impetus for carers and families to improve their quality of life and ensure that the rights and dignity of the person are respected.

CHAPTER 4

Benefits of Coping Strategies for People with Dementia, Carers and Families

The use of coping strategies introduces insightful responses and practices which can improve the experience and confidence of persons with dementia and carers, as well as the relationship with family members and friends. It also provides an increased opportunity to effect changes in the management of care and daily routines of personal care delivery.

For persons with dementia, their partners, families and carers, the adoption of dementia coping strategies will have the following advantages:

- Build resilience to deal with severe behavioural conditions and to manage the pressures or expectations from the person, carer and families.
- Have a better insight which enables a comforting response that helps to cope with the challenges of delivering daily care.
- Capable of practically managing their caring role, which includes handling new situations and other behavioural changes that may occur.
- Provide for the understanding and active acceptance of the person's dementia condition in order to get on with life in a positive and meaningful way.

- Acquire skills that could lead to the recognition of triggers of behaviour, or to deal with new challenges as the dementia progresses.
- Reduce incidents of emotional and physical fatigue, and be better able to deal with the burden of care and feelings of stress.
- Better able to adjust to the changes in lifestyle so as to improve their health and wellbeing.
- Increase carers' self-confidence, improve their self-esteem, and enable them to feel positive about themselves and their future.
- Improve the quality of life of the patient throughout all stages of the dementia pathway.
- Provide the opportunity for active involvement of family members in care delivery.

For health and social care professionals, coping strategies are likely to provide and re-enforce understanding of dementia care within a cultural and faith context. It will also enable professionals to better identify resource and support systems for people with dementia, their carers and families.

CHAPTER 5

Design of Suitable Coping Strategies for Carers

Behavioural changes and challenges are common conditions of people with dementia, and the experience of carers and families. This may be further aggravated by the stage of the dementia and type of dementia.

Within the homecare environment and existing dementia condition there are general and specific coping strategies that can be employed in order to provide:

(i) A level and quality of care that will ensure the comfort, safety and dignity of the person.
(ii) Better safeguarding of the person.
(iii) Improved management and delivery of long-term care needs.
(iv) Opportunities that empower carers to cope with all aspects of their care delivery.
(v) Creation of a more conducive and relaxing homecare environment.

There are a number of general guidelines to be considered that underline the approach to behavioural problems and the choice of suitable coping strategies to adopt:

(i) There is no standard or uniform experience or capability of being a carer.

(ii) Carers and families need to recognise and understand the likely situations that trigger behavioural problems and experiences.

(iii) While seeking to understand or determine the reason behind particular behaviours, finding a rational explanation may prove difficult.

(iv) Carers also need to understand that there are no prescribed or tested ways of dealing with behavioural problems, but that certain strategies can be helpful in dealing with specific behaviours.

(v) Carers must take steps to recognise the risk of harm to their patient or others and where there is considerable distress for the patient or themselves.

(vi) Whatever types of behaviour the person may display, every opportunity should be taken to give reassurance and comfort to the individual; for example, the person with dementia may be worried, or other things may not be real to the person.

(vii) Carers should recognise the difficulty in reasoning and not attempt to re-orientate the views or concerns of the person, but instead provide an explanation that might be acceptable and lots of reassurance.

(viii) While prompting may be employed to get a positive response from the person, this may change to a situation of non-compliance and later resistive care.

(ix) It is important for carers to be aware that contradiction often increases anxiety and confusion, and that the thought patterns of those with dementia are often fixed and cannot process contradiction or criticism.

(x) Some behavioural problems may require specialised help, advice or support obtained from medical, health or social care professionals.

CHAPTER 6

Introduction to Dementia Carers Coping Strategies

Coping strategies can be seen as the application of a set of actions, practices or responses in order to deal with recurring or developing care situations, finding solutions to particular problems, or coping and/or handling difficult or challenging behaviours.

For dementia carers and families, the use of coping strategies is aimed at:

(a) Providing a supportive framework in caring situations.
(b) Developing or practicing new or different approaches for dealing with difficult or challenging behaviours.
(c) Devising means of coping with stressful, emotionally disturbed or uncontrollable situations or experiences.
(d) Solving or finding solutions to particular dementia care-related issues and problems.

Practices employed in coping strategies

Various approaches, practices and styles may be employed by carers and families as coping strategies. These include:

- Avoid being rational and objective when dealing with the person. It may be necessary to enter into the person's reality.
- Avoid being argumentative, or seeking to engage not disagree with the person.
- Creating new routines or changing the way of doing things.
- Seeking support, such as emotional support from family and carers/peer groups.
- Engaging in activities that are relaxing and calming, such a meditation.
- Adjusting or managing expectations by adjusting to various outcomes in their caring role.
- Dealing with resentment, guilt or self-blame by avoiding feeling resentful of the additional responsibility and guilty for what is perceived as 'lack of empathy/compassion'.
- Change mind-set to desensitise and accept the role as carer.
- Physical recreation, such as regular exercises, including stretching exercises, meditating and other relaxation techniques.
- Respite care, or taking regular time out from the caring role for a few hours to a few days.

CHAPTER 7

Approach to Dementia Carers' Coping Strategies and Practices

Dementia often occurs as different types, with varying degrees of severity and in various stages, affecting individuals of different ages. With dementia there may also be individuals with mental health problems, medical conditions both chronic and acute, and with low, medium and high intensity care and support needs.

Hence the care of people with dementia may pose special difficulties and challenges for carers and families.

It is usual to find that the patient's condition declines and they become increasingly dependent or display changes in personality. Being unable to comprehend the nature of their dementia, they sometimes become un-cooperative and resentful of the carer.

Understanding the nature and impact of dementia changes and behavioural challenges on families is the first step towards the design and application of suitable coping strategies.

Coping strategies will need to be planned and implemented with a specific focus on the needs and in support of:

(a) **Dementia person:** feelings, mood, existing health or medical condition.

(b) **Dementia care:** dealing with specific behavioural problems of dementia conditions, quality of care, attainment of care goals and outcomes.

(c) **Carers:** role and responsibilities, needs, health and welfare considerations.

(d) **Families:** expectations, family value system, ethnic/cultural sensitivities.

(e) **Homecare environment:** current living and home environment

The design of coping strategies should also take into consideration:

- General approach or essential guidelines for use of coping strategies.
- Common triggers of dementia behavioural disturbances.
- Targeted strategies for dealing with specific behaviours or conditions.
- Planned or expected care outcomes for the person with dementia, their carer and families.

SECTION III

Understanding and Managing the Symptoms of Dementia

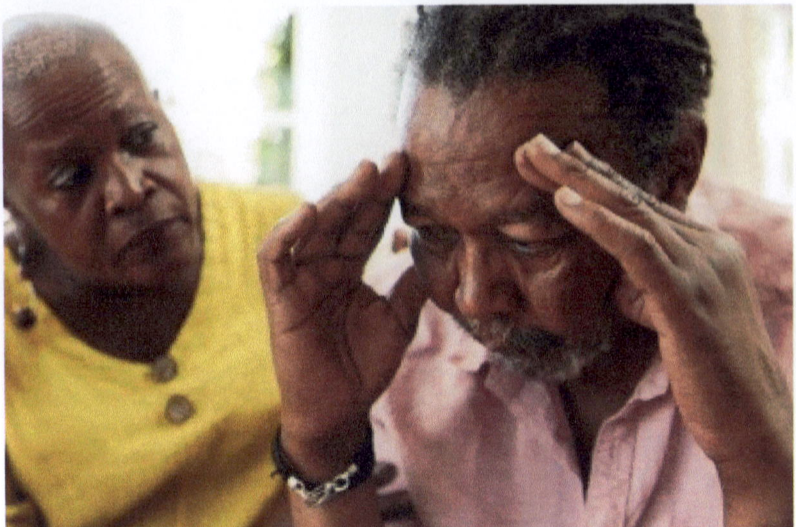

CHAPTER 8

Cognitive Impairments, Behavioural Manifestations and Functional Disabilities (Symptoms) in People with Dementia

Caring for people with dementia poses many challenges. As the disease progresses, personality and behavioural changes often occur. Challenging or concerning behaviour is used to describe behaviour that interferes with a person's daily life. It is considered one of the most difficult issues facing carers and families when caring at home.

These are in the nature of the behavioural, psychological and physical changes (symptoms) in people with dementia or Alzheimer's that present the greatest test for carers and families alike.

The following symptoms listed below can be broadly classified as:

(a) Behavioural manifestations;
(b) Cognitive impairment and;
(c) Functional disabilities/limitations.

These are some of the different ways people can be affected with dementia. The degree to which they are experienced will also differ between individuals.

Among the many changes/symptoms include:

(i) **Catastrophic reaction/high expressed emotion and rapid changes in mood:** over-reaction to trivial matters, which may result in weeping, screaming or unreasonable accusations.

(ii) **Repetitive/compulsive behaviour:** compulsion to follow relatives or staff asking the same questions over and over.

(iii) **Hoarding:** hoarding all sort of items for safekeeping; often accusing others of stealing their precious possessions.

(iv) **Loss of inhibition/inappropriate/impulsive behaviour:** loss of inhibitions and the consequent lack of awareness of the rules of appropriate behaviour.

(v) **Aggressiveness/anger and threatening behaviour:** physical (pushing, hitting) or verbal (abusive language)

(vi) **Paranoia/suspicions and delusions:** often suspicious of individuals and neighbours, they imagine that people are plotting against them. Also being suspicious of family.

(vii) **Wandering behaviour:** wandering manifests as pacing, lapping, walking and shadowing others, leaving safe areas unsupervised and getting lost when unaccompanied; leaving a safe environment or intruding in inappropriate places.

(viii) **Restlessness and fidgeting:** pacing and fidgeting, which this could be due to thirst, pain, medication side effects or even boredom, stress, noise, lack of exercises.

(ix) **Non-verbal agitation** (kicking, screaming, shouting, hitting): calling out continuously or weeping and whimpering for extended periods of time. (Sometimes this behaviour is a result of brain damage or hallucinations, and medical assistance may be required).

(x) **Sundowning:** an end-of-day confusion and restlessness that manifests as dusk approaches. Those affected may go into a heightened state of aggression or fearfulness, or they may suffer from delusions or paranoia and may begin pacing or wandering.

(xi) **Memory loss/difficulty paying attention:** (forgetting words or substituting inappropriate words)

(xii) **Misplacing things in inappropriate places**

(xiii) **Difficulty performing simple/familiar or routine tasks**

(xiv) **Problems in speaking, reading, writing and understanding**

(xv) **Loss of self-confidence:** this may show as apathy or disinterest in their usual activities.

(xvi) **Delusions:** unusual beliefs not based on reality

(xvii) **Hallucinations:** hearing or seeing things which are not real

(xviii) **Movement/physical weakness and slowness:** difficulty in movement or limited mobility

(xix) **Reduced mental sharpness and quickness:** reduced thinking speed

(xx) **Anxiety and agitation:** may feel anxious or agitated; may become restless, causing a need to move around or pace, or become upset in certain places or when focused on specific details.

(xxi) **Mental confusion:** getting 'muddled' when completing tasks and losing track of conversation.

(xxii) **Sleep disturbance:** sleep early during the day and can experience restless nights with nightmares.

(xxiii) **Bladder and bowel problems:** such as constipation and bladder and bowel incontinence.

(xxiv) **Impairment of co-ordination:** some types of dementia may lead to coordination problems, meaning a person cannot manage controlled movements; for example, when eating meals or dressing.

(xxv) **Falls:** people with dementia are at risk of falls because their sense of balance and ability to react quickly may be reduced, along with their memory and judgement.

(xxvi) **Difficulty in eating and drinking:** may find eating and drinking difficult for a range of reasons; for example, they may not recognise the food in front of them, they may find it hard to use a knife and fork or to chew or swallow food. Some may be at risk of choking because they have difficulty swallowing.

(xxvii) **Aphasia/dysphasia:** many people with dementia have difficulties with speech and language.

(xxviii) **Visual impairment:** problems interpreting what they see or recognising people or objects.

(xxix) **Impaired memory:** confabulations and intrusions in memory.

(xxx) **Dependence in relation to activities of daily living/self-care:** bathing, eating and toileting.

(xxxi) **Difficulty with balance and judging distance.**

The above changes in personality and behaviour (symptoms) are commonly observed in individuals with Alzheimer's disease, vascular dementia, dementia with Lewy bodies, fronto-temporal dementia and mild cognitive impairment.

CHAPTER 9

Common Triggers to Challenging Behaviours

People with dementia, particular of moderate to severe stages, may exhibit a range of behaviours that are often regarded as unpredictable, intense, irrational, disruptive, compulsive or even abusive. Sometimes problematic behaviours are caused by changes in the brain as the dementia progresses, and sometimes by triggers in the environment. Triggers may include:

(a) Problems with remembering and performing everyday activities are the most prominent symptoms. Many people with dementia also suffer from changes in mood, which can result in less motivation to perform their usual activities or a lack of interest in things around them.

(b) Anxiety about ordinary things, which may be exhibited by asking questions and repeating information about once-familiar events, or constantly attending to things which are not required or seeking explanations to things that are not real.

(c) Confusion about tasks that used to be routine, but may feel overwhelming.

(d) Frequent agitation may occur as people become less able to interpret their environment and control or express their feelings.

(e) Loss of ability to express themselves, as well as a diminished ability to communicate and eventually understand their feelings.

Triggers of dementia-related behaviours

It is important for carers and families to understand that individual behaviours are secondary conditions of the dementia disease process, and can occur throughout various stages of the disease.

There are many situations that act as triggers of dementia behaviours and that carers and family members should be made aware of in order to control or avoid such behaviours.

Sometimes problematic behaviours are caused by changes in the brain as the dementia progresses, and sometimes by changes in their environment. There are also psychological and medical triggers.

Such triggers may include:

- The environment: too hot or cold, too quiet or too busy.
- Inappropriate environment: noisy, crowded room, chaotic gathering.
- Interactions: feeling rushed, not understanding words, not feeling listened to.
- Lack of activity: boredom may prompt the patient to look for something to do.
- Too much stimulation: loud music, frantic environment.

- Frustration: not being able to perform tasks that could be done before.
- Physical discomfort: illness, side effects of medication.
- Physical discomfort: pain, hunger, thirst, needing the toilet.
- Unfamiliar surroundings: new furniture, renovation in facility, new to residential care.
- Altered circadian rhythm: confusion caused by disrupted sleep.
- Disorientation: searching for a familiar face or urge to go 'home' or go to 'work'.
- Ourselves: personality, personal history and experiences, habits, likes and dislikes.
- Not being to find something: such as a lost wallet, walking stick or handbag.
- Dehydration.
- Fatigue.
- Insomnia.
- Depression.
- Fear/feeling frightened.
- Frustration.
- Visuals and hallucinations.
- Restlessness.
- Anxiety or agitation.

CHAPTER 10

Recognising Situations that Trigger Dementia-related Behaviours

Situations that trigger dementia behaviours may be broadly classified as:

(i) Being overwhelmed or confused by the physical or social environment

The behaviour of the individual may need to be examined as a reaction to the surroundings. Key environmentally-based factors that may contribute to challenging behaviours are:

- Physical environment: this may be unfamiliar or too complex understand.
- Physical environment: the home may be cluttered, distracting or difficult to sort out.
- Social environment: complex communication may cause feelings of confusion, fear and anxieties. It may also be strained and unhelpful and contribute to resistance.
- Difficulty in interpreting environmental signals and responding appropriately.
- Having unfamiliar people around.

(ii) Situations that cause emotional upheaval or disturbance

- Presence of someone that causes upset.
- Thinking or missing someone who was close or dear to them in the past.
- Wanting to communicate or visit individuals who are no longer alive.

(iii) Trying to do things that cause frustration or dissatisfaction

- Sources of stress in the environment, such as daily activities, changes in routines or new situations.
- Memory impairment also affects behaviour and daily performance capabilities of the individual.
- Unable to understand or to explain.
- Instructions may be overwhelming.
- Activities that may be too complex or unfamiliar.
- Poor coordination in dealing with some activities.
- Feel frustrated because of not being able to communicate his/her needs.
- Not being able to hear what is being said and continually asking for information to be repeated, adding to their own frustrations.

(iv) Situations that may trigger agitation or restlessness

- Feelings of fear and insecurity.
- Inability to understand what is required to be done.
- Feelings of loneliness, isolation or frustration.

- Changes in social environment, for example meeting new or unfamiliar people.
- Not being able to communicate his/her needs.
- Lacks ability to perform certain functions.

(v) Situations that may trigger wandering

- Lack of activity, stimulation or boredom.
- Too much stimulation: loud music, frantic environment.
- Physical discomfort: illness, side effects of medication.
- Disorientation: searching for a familiar face or urge to go 'home' or go to 'work'.
- The belief that they can do things which they are not capable of doing.
- Believing that they have to do things or go to some event that may not be real.
- Unrealistic worrying about wanting to visit someone or someplace, or check on things that are not real.
- Frustration at being unable to perform tasks that could be done before.
- Obsession action of going to the kitchen or to the door for no obvious reason.
- Unfamiliar surroundings: new furniture, renovation in facility, new to residential care.

(vi) Triggers that may cause hallucinations or false perceptions of realities

- Confusion in the way some things or someone is perceived.

- Images and noises from radio and television may be perceived as a real persons or someone who is not there.
- Inability to recognise a spouse or partner and the house where there the patient is living.
- Inadequate lighting that makes visual objects and cues less clear.

(vii) Situations that trigger hoarding

- A response to feelings of isolation.
- Link to anxiety or fear of losing something.
- Response to memory loss.

(viii) Medical or mental health conditions

- Behaviours may also be the result of underlying medical or mental health problems, such as infection or lack of sleep.
- Medications that may contribute to decreased cognitive function.

(ix) Common triggers of sundowning

The term 'sundowning' or 'sundown syndrome' refers to an end-of-day confusion and restlessness that manifests as dusk approaches. It affects people living with Alzheimer's disease and other forms of dementia. Sundowning causes behavioural problems that begin to occur as the sun is setting.

Those affected may go into a heightened state of aggression or fearfulness from delusions or paranoia, or begin pacing or wandering.

Sundowning may be triggered by:

- Other related trigger conditions such as delusion, confusion, disorientation or agitation.
- Unable to cope with stressful conditions.
- Poor lighting causing shadows may result in confusion, anxiety or fear.
- Fatigue: mental or physical exhaustion at the end of the day.
- Loss of purpose and sense of security.
- Wanting to go home.
- Wanting to visit a place or relative which does not exist.
- Mix up between day and night.
- Poor sleeping patterns.
- Unmet needs: thirsty, cold, hungry.
- Boredom.
- Stimulating drinks: coffee or alcohol.

(x) Inability to respond to carers' or family members' responses or expectations

- Condemning or pointing out failures or mistakes.
- Carers shouting or scolding the patient.
- Displaying anger or frustration towards the patient.
- Shouting or scolding the patient.

(xi) Triggers of repetition or repeated questioning

- Feeling separated or lonely.
- Feeling insecure or lost.
- Inability to express a need.

(xii) Situations that trigger anger and aggression

- Fear of a situation or a person that the patient finds threatening.
- Feeling lost or insecure.
- Fatigue or disruption of sleep pattern.
- Situations that are unfamiliar to the patient.
- Feelings of pain or physical discomfort.

Behaviour therefore has a profound effect on the carer and family members, mainly because it increases the carers' burden and stress and ultimately the quality of life. It remains for carers and family members to find ways to minimize or manage behaviours through eliminating or modifying all triggers and contributory factors.

CHAPTER 11

Managing and Coping with Challenging Behaviours

Caring for people with dementia poses many challenges. As the disease progresses, personality and behavioural changes often occur.

Challenging or concerning behaviour is used to describe behaviour that interferes with a person's daily life. It is considered one of the most difficult issues facing family carers at home.

Challenging behaviour is distressing for both the person exhibiting the behaviour and for those that care for them. It is important to try and understand why the person is behaving in a particular way and remember that it is the behaviour that is challenging and not the person.

There are times when some people with dementia become agitated and display other unwanted behaviours. Try to find out what is behind the behaviour, such as sickness, sadness, environmental factors, fatigue, depression, or provocation.

(i) Approach in a calm, respectful manner.

(ii) It is best not to touch the person by leading or holding the arms, as this aggravates the situation. Instead talk in a consoling and empathetic manner, offer your arm and say,

"Here, take my arm, let's go to the dining room/bedroom/ veranda."

(iii) Try not to over-react even if the behaviour is embarrassing. Remember that it is the illness causing the behaviour.

(iv) Avoid arguing. Remember the person is not deliberately trying to upset you. Their logic and reasoning are impaired by the illness and it is up to you to comfort and reassure them.

(v) Be flexible. For example, if the behaviour is about a shower they don't want to have, leave this task for later when the person has calmed down.

(vi) Observe the person and what their body language is conveying. Give them time to calm down while offering solace.

(vii) Validate their feelings. If an elderly lady is very agitated and asks you whether you have seen her mother, it is no use pointing out to her that she is dead. Go along with her and say something like, "No, I haven't seen her. Was she a great cook? What did she cook that you loved?"

(viii) Be mindful and 'in the moment'. If you are talking to the person and your thoughts are elsewhere there is a good chance you won't get the best result. Often your body language and demeanour will speak louder than your words. Use a soft tone of voice and some physical touch, if appropriate, to add emphasis to the communication.

(ix) Offer a distraction such as a walk or a game.

For person-centred care

1. Implement individually tailored, flexible routines.
2. Recognize that it is important to get to know the person beyond the diagnosis.
3. Remember that nutrition and hydration are important factors.
4. Aim to reduce anti-psychotic medication wherever possible.
5. Strive to anticipate concerning behaviours.
6. Schedule activities that promote creativity and satisfaction.
7. Provide guidance and reassurance with compassionate overtones.
8. Implement behaviour management strategies with an emphasis on dignity and respect.
9. Gentle touch and physical contact is important and can reduce fear and anxiety.
10. Ensure there is a collaborative partnership between carer and patient.

Understanding what may be causing the challenging behaviour and learning how to respond to it will enable carers to take control of situations when they arise and diminish the occurrence of the behaviour.

CHAPTER 12

Strategies for Coping with Specific Dementia Behaviours

Coping strategies for common dementia behaviours:

(i) Dealing with aggression (verbal and physical), anger and abuse

Aggressive behaviour is probably one of the principal conditions of dementia. Aggression may be linked to internal factors, such as depression and pain, and external factors, including quality of carer, patient relationship and environmental factors.

In reducing or preventing aggression carers should endeavour to:

- Remove or eliminate all stressful situations.
- Try to recognise the cause of the behaviour.
- Be mindful of all aspects of the patient's personal care.
- Get the patient involved in various recreational activities, such as singing and painting.
- Allow the patient to cool down.
- Listen to the patient and avoid arguing or be confrontational.

- Try to reassure the patient by speaking slowly and with a reassuring voice.
- Try to redirect the patient's interest to change the focus away from the matter causing the aggression.
- Be aware of the patient's body language, expression and tone of voice.

ii Dealing with fear and agitation

When patients become agitated they may be difficult to handle as they are not in control of their emotions or not able to understand. It is important for the carer to take into account the patient's current state and beliefs by:

- Staying calm at all times.
- Listening in a calm, affectionate, reassuring manner.
- Using verbal and non-verbal ways of reassuring the patient.
- Avoiding arguing/correcting/insisting that the patient is wrong or unreasonable.
- If the patient is threatening the physical safety of the carer, stepping back or leaving the scene.
- If the patient is harming himself/herself, holding the patient firmly with the minimal strength necessary to stop self-harm.
- Try to understand and address the patient's emotional need.
- Use of soft, soothing music may be helpful.
- Seeking to distract the patient may sometimes work.

iii When a patient is delusional and believes in other realities

- Carers must at all times avoid arguing or trying to explain or correct the patient.
- Avoid a situation where the patient gets upset.
- Try to understand the underlying emotions, the realities and concerns of the patient, and address and reconcile with them.
- Carers may find it necessary to join in with the imaginary realities of the patient.

iv Dealing with agitation or restlessness

- Reduce or eliminate feelings of uncertainty or confusion by keeping to routines.
- Pay attention to ways of communication by using short and simple statements.
- Create tranquil, calming surroundings by reducing stress and playing soft music.
- Avoid asking questions or seeking answers.
- Avoid rebuking the patient.
- Seek to reassure and comfort the patient.

v Dealing with dementia-related wandering

- Listen carefully and be 'present' or they will notice. In other words, don't underestimate patients.
- Try to re-direct or distract the patient's interest or attention with another activity.

- Avoid correcting the patient's perception of reality.
- Approach calmly and make patients feel that you understand whatever they are going through by speaking slowly and serenely.
- Reassure the patient as to where he or she is at present and return to routine as soon as possible.
- Help the patient to connect with familiar items, place or objects.
- Distract the patient with another activity to reduce anxiety.
- Show concern, and make the patient feel safe and secure by agreeing with what is being said.
- If the patient is aggressive, back away and come back later.

vi Dealing with sundowning

- Choose a suitable room for relaxation.
- Provide bright lighting in room to help identify objects.
- Try to keep the patient calm when agitation occurs.
- Play soft and relaxing music.
- Keep the person engaged in activities he/she enjoys during the day.
- Avoid giving the patient highly stimulating drinks such as coffee.
- Offer the patient reassurance, and reminisce to provide distraction.
- Exercise, dance or waltz to music in the mornings to get the blood flowing.

- Keep familiar things and comfort objects like dolls, favourite blankets, soft toys, family photographs close by.

vii Dealing with hallucinations

- Reduce or get rid of clutter in the home so as to reduce confusion.
- Increase lighting in rooms frequented by the patient as this may reduce stress.
- Remove or get rid of things or items in the home that might appear confusing or be perceived as real people or events.
- Label rooms, drawers or cupboards using suitable colours and/or pictures to reduce confusion.
- Observe what the patient is doing or looking at and what might be causing the mis-perception.

viii Dealing with hoarding

- Gradually remove items and try to get the patient to agree.
- Attempt to reorganise and clear out items.
- Show compassion and avoid using logic to get the patient to understand.
- Try getting the patient to agree if they have the ability or capacity to understand or reason.

ix Dealing with repetition or repeated questioning

- Give the patient something to do or to occupy his/her time.

- Seek to reassure the patient and to convey a feeling of empathy and warmth.
- Try to detect and respond to the emotion behind each question.
- Seek to distract the patient with activities he/she enjoys doing.
- Speak calmly and try to answer the question each time.

CHAPTER 13

Understanding and Managing Types of Dementia-related Behaviours

All behaviours have meaning

People's behaviour, whatever form it takes, is very often an attempt to express something which they are unable to articulate verbally. The way in which people with dementia act may be in response to a particular situation, or reflect a need they have, hence the need to try to understand what is happening and why it is happening before working out what to do.

Managing behaviour is a process that guides carers to change their actions within a specific time frame.

Assessment of behaviour

A considered assessment may give carers and families an understanding of the meaning of the behaviour. What may have happened a few hours ago, or the previous day, for example, will help to identify early symptoms or triggers so that they can alter their course in the future. A behaviour can be considered appropriate or inappropriate. This is often related to social and/or cultural ideas.

Carers should identify the behaviour patterns in terms of frequency, such as every half hour, all day long, only when family visits, and how long the behaviour lasts. Be objective in the description of the individual's actions, and avoid vague terms such as 'annoying' or 'strange' behaviour. Different people can act in different ways, even in the same situation. This can reflect their experiences and their interpretation of the situation.

Challenging behaviours

Challenging behaviours refer to inappropriate, vocal and sometimes hostile behaviour. Whether it is intentional or not, it is a concern that impacts on everyone's quality of life.

There are many factors that influence behaviours in dementia care. These include:

- Functional losses, handicap.
- Physical health: pain, discomfort and/or infection.
- Cognitive deficit deterioration

Other possible reasons for challenging or problem behaviours

Sometimes the cause of problem behaviour is not related to any of the above. Instead, poor day-to-day interactions between the individual and carer/family and friends may prompt the undesirable behaviour through misunderstanding, miscommunication and unnoticed upsets, such as:

- Ineffective use of discipline: harsh reaction to crisis, staff inconsistencies.
- Ignoring or rewarding poor behaviour.

- Perceived escalation of triggers from the point of view of dementia person and others.
- Overlooked body language.
- Guilt-inducing message from family and/or friends.
- Antagonism between the dementia person and others.
- Environmental factors.
- Conflicting instructions: too many, too quick, too vague.

Examples of challenging behaviours

These include:

- Physical aggression.
- Verbal aggression.
- Wandering.
- Responding to visual hallucinations.
- Being repetitive.

Managing disruptive behaviour

There is no 'one size fits all' solution. Non-pharmacological interventions are the preferred approach. Use strategies that increase positive behaviour and reduce negative behaviour, such as:

- **Exude a positive attitude.** First, you need to have a positive attitude and be smiling and upbeat. A person with dementia takes cues from you, so if you are smiling, happy and upbeat, there is a good chance the person will be too.

- **Try to refocus and redirect attention.** Despite everyone's best efforts, you might just sense that the problem behaviour is escalating. It is best to stop what you are doing, and help the person with dementia to calm down by refocusing and redirecting their attention.
- **Identify 'stop' behaviours.** Everyone needs to know what works best to stop these unpleasant behaviours. That is why knowing the person is critical.
- **Never argue.** Another must is NEVER argue with a person who has dementia. This is the one thing that will set them off most. Instead enter his or her reality.
- **Ask for help.** Everyone likes to feel useful. Make sure you tell the residents that you need their help.
- **Focus on feelings.** Remember it's all about feelings when interacting with a person who has dementia.
- **Give compliments.** Besides saying hello and smiling, you can be complimentary. All people tend to be in a better mood if you say something nice about them. Learn what makes the person with dementia tick, and how to make him/her feel good about him/herself.

Managing aggressive behaviour

Providing care for a person with aggressive behaviour can be extremely challenging. If the person is rude or aggressive, it is the carer's job to find ways to manage the situation and maintain a peaceful environment. This does not mean that the disgruntled person should be punished or scolded for his/her behaviour.

When approaching and interacting with a person who is obviously angry or upset, carers and family members should:

- **Approach slowly.** Use slow and calm movements so you don't add tension to the situation.
- **Get to their level.** Remain at eye level with the person. If they are in a wheelchair sit beside them, don't stand or hover above them.
- **Give them privacy.** Invite the resident to speak in a more private setting.
- **Mirror facial expressions.** If the forehead is scrunched up, scrunch yours up. Mirroring facial expressions is a form of validation that shows a person that you see them as well as hear them.
- **Validate their feelings.** Tell them that you see that they are upset, frustrated, or angry. Validation is one of the quickest ways to de-escalate a situation.
- **Give them space.** Sometimes a carer will want to keep an eye on the person that is aggressive or manipulative, however, providing space for the him/her to calm down is important and gives them an opportunity to reflect on the situation.

Reactions to avoid

Carers and family members should never:

- **Punish**. For example, sending a resident to their room or taking certain privileges away from them.
- **Argue.** Arguing will make the situation worse.
- **Use negative body language.** Don't point fingers, cross arms or put hands on hips.

- **Publicise bad behaviour.** Never discuss a person's behaviour publicly to other residents or in the hallways where other staff and residents can hear.
- **Withhold care.** Denying care is neglect and, in severe cases, can even be considered cruelty.

Increasing positive behaviour

- Draw on remaining skills/capabilities regardless of level of cognitive status.
- Use social reinforcement like smiles, a caring attitude, acceptance and praise.
- Listen attentively.
- Offer one-to-one social interaction.
- Distract with music of choice, outings, pets, games.
- Reward patients with social attention or food/drink (for example, a cup of tea) whenever you see them demonstrating kindness, patience, or when smiling.

Steps to reduce disruptive behaviour

- Seek staff support and cooperation.
- Engage family cooperation: more visits, videos from family and grandchildren.
- Massage therapy.
- Aromatherapy.
- Reward patients with social attention or food/drink (for example, a cup of tea) whenever you see them demonstrating kindness, patience, or when smiling.

- Always remember (and remind others) that it is the behaviour that is challenging and not the person.

Positive reinforcement interventions

Tuning into desirable behaviours is an intervention that can increase positive behaviours and decrease negative behaviours:

(i) Remember individuals with dementia want to preserve their independence and dignity.

(ii) Observe the patient closely and, when the opportunity arises, comment on positive behaviour.

(iii) Describe the approved behaviour: "This is wonderful, Mary, please show me how you do it!"

(iv) Be enthusiastic and sincere.

(v) Smile and maintain eye contact with patient at all times.

(vi) During activities and conversations, and whilst doing chores or playing games, reward the individual with social approval and attention – asking questions related to the activity, for example – and complimenting them on performance as above.

(vii) Take an interest in what the individual is doing. Persons with dementia usually appreciate your attention and this can be a powerful motivator.

(viii) Initially attend to patients immediately and often when reinforcing positive behaviour.

(ix) Seek to learn about the person, or try to understand the person so as to better connect with them.

(x) When dealing with resistive behaviour, first initiate the thought, give the person a moment, then have the individual participate in the action.

(xi) Seek to encourage a nurturing and supportive environment to help the person feel happy and safe.

Remember that non-verbal behavior can convey a great deal of meaning to patients. For example, sitting by the patient or standing nearby, touching, joining in activities or smiling.

CHAPTER 14

Dealing with Diminished or Lack of Capacity and Functional Disability

There are often progressive and significantly diminished capacity and functional disabilities that occur for people with dementia, and which can affect their independence, quality of life, and ability to live safely at home, particularly if living alone. This may result in neglect or difficulty in maintaining personal care and hygiene, such as bathing, dressing, grooming, difficulty with taking medications, and preparing and eating adequate meals.

Some of the cognitive abilities required to perform functional tasks, adequate long and short-term memory, and appropriate insight and safety awareness may be diminished or lost in cases of moderate to severe dementia

People with dementia often lack the ability to plan and execute simple or complex tasks, which may require the ability to integrate various cognitive skills, such as making a pot of tea.

Lack of specific forms of capacity and diminished functional disability in persons with dementia

Lack of capacity can be broadly classified with reference to some of the following forms:

- **Financial capacity.** Lacks capacity or ability to make simple or complex financial decision. For example, operating a bank account.
- **Functional capacity.** Lacks capacity to plan or execute simple or complex tasks. For example, making a cup of tea.
- **Mental capacity.** Lacks capacity to make their own decisions.
- **Health and welfare capacity.** Lacks ability to make future health and welfare decisions.
- **Daily living or independent living.** Lacks capacity to perform simple daily personal care tasks. For example, getting dressed.
- **Mobility.** Lacks the ability to drive a vehicle
- **Legal.** Lacks the ability or cognitive capability to create or enter into a legal transaction.

Each form of diminished or limited capacity/ability will attract a specific form of intervention or approach, including referral to a particular source or action to be taken.

Strategies for coping with diminished capacity and functional disabilities

Whatever the patient's cognitive level or functional capabilities, rehabilitative strategies can be offered to facilitate some learning. This would include simplifying tasks, establishing routines, practicing tasks through repetition and practice, and providing task-specific training.

The overall aim is to strengthen the patient's functioning capabilities, which can be done through:

- Treatment of underlying conditions.
- Physical and occupational therapy.
- Assistive devices.
- Use of practical aids, such as hearing or visual aids, and reminders.
- Activities that involve brain training.
- Skills training, development or rehabilitation.

SECTION IV

Cultural and Ethnic Considerations in Dementia Care

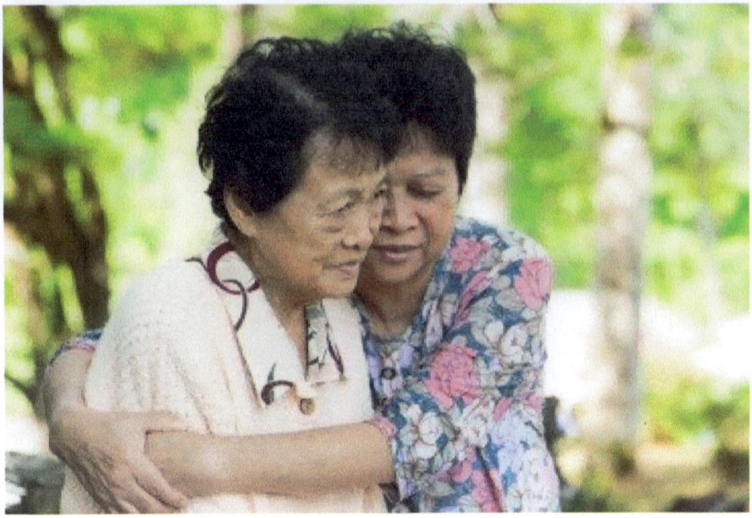

CHAPTER 15

Strategies for Supporting Carers and Families

There are various forms of behavioural changes that occur as part of the dementia condition. Coping with these changes and challenges has a major impact on the physical, mental and emotional health and wellbeing of carers and families. Dementia carers and families will be expected to practice ways in managing the various issues in their caring role.

Issues regarding the caring role of dementia carers

There are many issues to be considered by carers and family members when dealing with dementia person care involving severe behavioural challenges. These include:

- Managing and coping with specific forms of behaviours.
- Coping with the physical and emotional demands of caring.
- Creation of a safe and comfortable environment.
- Addressing the physical, mental and emotional health needs of the carer.
- Preserving the dignity and self-respect of the person.
- Seeking to enhance the quality of the person cared for.

(a) Addressing the physical, mental and emotional health of carers

Carers and family members may regularly experience feelings of guilt, anger and frustration, which may be extreme and internal at times. Such feelings are often the result of:

- Loss of companionship or meaningful relationship with their love ones.
- Changes in personality and behaviour.
- Anger or upsets with the patient's behaviour.
- Feelings of guilt about the way the patient's care needs are delivered.
- Having to undertake caring duties that are culturally sensitive.
- Failure to get help from family members.
- The need to be removed from the caring situation.
- Not seeing an end to their caring role.
- Feelings made worse by the carer's poor health.

(b) Coping strategy for dealing with mental and emotional needs of carers

- Carers should attempt to define the problem, explore possible causes, and think about ways to overcome/deal with it.
- Carers should try to make their caring role a positive experience for their patients and the families.
- Carers should find ways to actively involve family members in managing and the delivery of care.

- They should actively find ways of managing their stressful conditions. This may be done by:

(i) Learning as much as possible about dementia.

(ii) Trying different solutions in order to find the one that best works for them.

(ii) Trying to be realistic about what can be expected of them.

(iii) Paying attention to matters of health with regards to sleep, diet and regular exercise.

- Carers should seek comfort and practical assistance by attending carers' support group meetings with families, other carers and friends.
- As much as possible, carers should try to develop a new interest aside from their caring responsibilities.
- Carers should undertake activities that are enjoyable or beneficial.
- They should avail themselves of regular respite breaks.

CHAPTER 16

Gender Considerations - Caring for a Person with Dementia

Addressing the physical, mental and emotional needs of male carers.

The quality of life for male carers is mostly expressed through the experience of their physical, work, social and home environment. This is revealed in the nature of their communications, relationships and daily interactions. It has become increasingly common to find male carers attending to the care and support needs of a partner or parent. Thrust into a caring role, there are issues and challenges that directly impact every aspect of the male carer's relationships, communications and social life, which need to be addressed.

While many of the experiences of caring for a person with dementia are common to both male and female carers, there are issues that largely feature in the experience of the male carer.

Issues for male carers

There are a number of issues that shape the experience of male carers. Among these are:

- Adjusting to changes in lifestyle.
- Handling the caring role, including new routines.

- Changed relationship with the person they care for.
- Difficulty engaging with the cared for person.
- Coping with the physical and emotional demands of caring.
- Difficulty in acceptance of the role as carer.
- Homecare environment no longer relaxing.
- Lacks opportunity for physical exercise.
- Lack of companionship or meaningful relationship with a loved one.
- Dealing with changes in personality and behaviour.
- Dealing with resentment, guilt or self-blame.
- Feeling of isolation and social exclusion
- Lack of empathy.
- Undertaking caring roles that are culturally sensitive.
- Not seeing the end into the caring role.
- Need to be removed from the caring situation.
- Lack of contact with friends, family and the community.
- Feeling or the perception of being alone in the world, even when people are around.
- Low self-esteem.
- Compassion fatigue characterised by emotional and physical exhaustion that diminishes ability to feel empathy resulting from the constant demands of caring.
- Feelings of irritability, anger and guilt.

Among the many contributory factors include:

i. Dwindling resources.
ii. Coping with certain aspects of personal care.

iii. Person cared for going through a difficult phase.

iv. Difficulty in accessing information, support and services.

v. Personal circumstances.

vi. Lack of essential knowledge and caring skills.

vii. Lack of support and help from other family members.

Strategies for coping with the mental and emotional needs of male carers

For the male carer, they should aim for the following:

i) Try to change how you think about yourself, your situation and the consequences it has on you.
ii) Try to make the caring role a positive experience.
iii) Strive to improve the experience and environment of you the carer.
iv) Manage stressful conditions.
v) Develop new interests.
vi) Have regular respite breaks.
vii) Seek comfort and practical assistance by attending a carers' support group.
viii) Invest in things that give you meaning and purpose in your life.
ix) Find ways to feel empowered, such as focusing on things you can control.
x) Ask for help and support from others.
xi) Seek to maintain your personal relationships.
xii) Pay attention to your health.

xiii) Be prepared for changes to occur over time. When this happens, try to adapt to the new situation or state of affairs.

xiv) Try to adapt your priorities and standards of achievement to your current abilities. If necessary, lower your expectations a little

xv) Pay attention to self-care habits, such as good nutrition, sleep, daily practice of relaxation (mindfulness or yoga), and nurturing activities.

xvi) Take one day at a time. While thinking about the future is normal, try and focus on the challenges of caring just one day at a time.

xvii) Discuss possible work options with your employer. Many employers offer flexible working arrangements.

xviii) Get someone to do your household chores. Ask a relative, or consider a local private service, or access help at your local council.

CHAPTER 17

Cultural and Ethnic Issues Influencing Dementia Care
Providing Culturally and Ethnically Appropriate Care

Cultural diversity and inclusion are important factors influencing the care for those with dementia. Providing culturally sensitive care is essential for supporting these individuals, their carers and families from diverse cultural backgrounds. It is therefore important for health and social care providers to understand and respond effectively to the multicultural and linguistic needs of family carers. Hence cultural competence is a critical requirement that is achieved through awareness and training of staff and with policies related to cultural diversity.

'Cultural diversity has many key dimensions: history, language, race, traditions, beliefs, ethnicity and ideas shared by a group of people. It determines how people see the world and their place in it.'

'Inclusion refers to the right of all those involved to participate and have equity in all aspects of life.'

'Cultural Competence is defined as a set of behaviours, attitudes, and practices that equip health and social care providers with the knowledge to deliver culturally appropriate care.'

Embracing cultural diversity and promoting inclusion are two aspects of cultural competence.'

A significant number of carers and families these days are from diverse cultural backgrounds, hence a 'one size fits all' approach is not effective.

From whatever background the person with dementia may come from the experience of dementia is going to be individual. Likewise, family carers are from a range of different backgrounds with their own experience on a personal level. Carers and families of persons with dementia tend to experience many similar behavioural and psychological symptoms, such as emotional and physical fatigue, stress, depression and social isolation. This, to a large extent, would indicate the social and healthcare needs, including support, information and advice.

Care sector workers, including health and social care professionals, also run the risk of introducing implicit and explicit biases, with unconscious beliefs and stereotypes of a particular group of people or cultures. These biases, whether intentional or not, can have profound effects on the quality of care provided and the resulting quality of life for persons with dementia and their families. This means finding positive ways of engaging with people living with dementia, their carers and families from specific communities – that is, support and services that are sensitive to and respectful of cultural, ethnic and religious differences.

To support cultural diversity, health and social care professionals need to acquire a level of cultural competence. Cultural competence is developed over time and includes self-awareness, guidance, training and experience.. Embracing cultural diversity means appreciating the differences in individuals from a variety of cultural and ethnic groups. A culture that celebrates cultural diversity and promotes inclusion must be interwoven into the care, activity and support plans for those with dementia, their carers and families.

Unfortunately, studies indicate that there are differences in the way carers and families from minority ethnic communities tend to access support and services Carers and families from African-Caribbean communities tend to have 'blended' families who are often involved in caring. Such communities are largely motivated by perceptions of 'duty', setting an example to children, religious or spiritual beliefs, family teachings and expectations. They often provide care in collectivist rather than individualistic caregiving systems. This determines the nature and level of interaction among families and friends involved in the caring role.

Another common feature is that such communities tend to make use of their local church support groups as a means of trying to avoid the stigma of cognitive impairment and behavioural changes. For many families, such groups provide an alternative to professional services They are more likely to delay and might avoid engaging with professionals from social care agencies or services in the uptake of formal support and services as long as possible.

The reasons for these discrepancies vary from differences in beliefs and practices, language barriers, non-adherence to treatments, differences in lifestyle, thinking style, philosophy of life and other traits.

Barriers faced in accessing support and services by ethnic minorities

There are many perceived barriers from recognising dementia, accessing social care, support and services, as well as from providing culturally appropriate care. These range from:

(i) Lack of awareness and knowledge of dementia.
(ii) Failure to recognise symptoms of dementia, coupled with the belief that the symptoms are part of the normal aging process.
(iii) Inability to recognise and accept the onset of dementia.
(iv) Spiritual and religious beliefs that add to the misconception of dementia.
(v) Language barriers, especially in older persons indicating linguistic needs are not met.
(vi) Lack of cultural 'fit' – that is, appropriateness of services provided may diminish the extent of family preference for accessing support.
(vii) Low service uptake/utilisation due to lack of knowledge, cultural and family beliefs.
(viii) Cultural norms and beliefs that contribute to the social stigma and shame faced by families may result in failure to discuss dementia openly with family members, or isolating the person from the community.
(ix) In some ethnic groups there is evidence of delay in seeking formal assessment until the person's condition (behaviour and other symptoms) becomes severe.
(x) Reluctance to discuss the psychological distress caused from caring at home.
(xi) Sense of duty, guilt, social pressures and cultural norms may have a negative effect on the caring role.
(xii) Difficulty in accessing health and social care.

Levels at which coping strategies targeting support and service users and providers can be effective

Among minority communities, and Asian communities in particular, there is a preference to deliver homecare instead of institutional care, hence the need to empower carers and families through training, information, advice, support and services. It also indicates that services will need to be provided at the community, health and social care and family network levels. This can best be done by:

- Promoting services through ethnic media.
- Increasing awareness of available services.
- Adapting or customising services to specific cultural needs of different ethnic groups.
- Building carers' and professional workers' capability to reflect on service delivery.
- Arranging and encouraging attendance at group meetings and discussions as a forum to discuss health and social care needs, and connect individuals to the right services.

Strategies for supporting racially and culturally diverse dementia care recipients, their carers and families

To deliver culturally appropriate care, the focus should be on maintaining and affirming cultural identity and knowledge. The coping strategies for dealing with people with dementia, their carers and families, require taking into consideration a number of approaches and practices relating to:

- Raising awareness about dementia to combat stigma.
- Relevant training and support in developing effective communication strategies to deliver individually tailored and culturally sensitive care.
- A recognition and response to carers' needs.

- Raising awareness of services among service users and providers through literacy and practical support.
- Improving information about services and access pathways.
- Improved engagement with people from racial, ethnic and cultural backgrounds in the development and delivery of culturally appropriate care services to facilitate understanding of dementia and improve access.

Compassionate communication

The need is to understand that beliefs and traditions are powerful forces in a person's life.

Patient behaviour can be based on misguided perceptions. For example, in some cultures nodding the head means acknowledging but not accepting what is being said. Therefore, do not make assumptions, even if the patient can speak English, and try to keep communication as simple as possible to avoid confusion and misinterpretation. Also, consider learning some key words in different languages to better communicate with patients.

Show empathy and interest

Demonstrate openness to exploring issues from the point of view of the patient's culture. Remember that there are many similarities as well as differences across cultures. Build on the similarities to help each other.

Eliminate prejudice

Be aware that prejudice is prevalent in most societies. It is essential to eliminate biases and discrimination and cultivate tolerance and compassion.

Engage volunteers

Find bilingual volunteers to help support patients from multicultural backgrounds. They will appreciate the opportunity to enjoy the company of someone who speaks their language and understands their culture.

Collaborate with relatives

Ask relatives for advice and involve them in decision-making.

Support religious and spiritual beliefs

Accept that religion, spirituality and beliefs may influence how patients behave.

Provide linguistic support

Provide translation services, radio podcasts and videos relevant to the cultural background of patients.

Cultural Leisure Activities

Foster relationships with community organisations relevant to the cultures at clubs, neighbourhood groups and carers' groups.

Cultural support in care plans

Develop care plans that are compatible with your patient's community affiliations. Their 'social profile' is perhaps the most important tool that can used to assess patients. This document should be compiled in collaboration with the patient, their relatives, activity staff and other allied health and social care providers.

SECTION V

Understanding the Dementia Care Environment

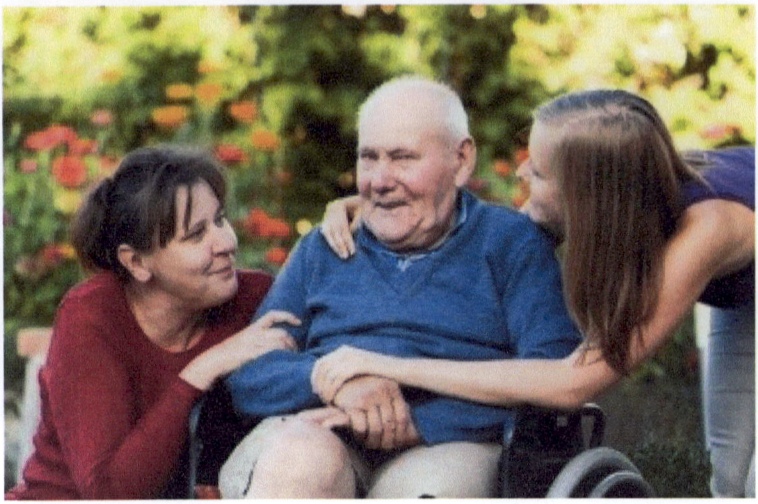

CHAPTER 18

Improving Dementia Persons Environment and Experience

The care and support needs of people with dementia are mainly provided and delivered as home-based care, community care, such as in residential care homes, and as respite care in the institutional care setting. However, family networks remain the cornerstone of dementia patient care delivery.

Most dementia patients continue to live with their families, and that care is usually delivered as a joint effort by adult members of the family. Individual family members may usually be involved with the caring and are often considered as the primary carer.

Against this background, it is important for carers and families to gain an understanding of the dementia care environment and how it may affect the behaviour of the person or the impact it may have on their role.

Understanding the environment also informs on the various health and social care services and ways of accessing services. This also covers health and welfare issues, and property and financial affairs that concern dementia patients. Issues regarding standards and quality of care, approach to care planning and delivery, support and resource for patients, are also key to understanding the overall dementia care and support environment.

The dementia care environment mainly consists of:

(i) The dementia physical environment, both indoor and outdoor.

(ii) The wider operating dementia care environment.

(iii) The dementia homecare environment.

(iv) Dementia institutional care environment.

(v) Dementia community care environment.

(a) Physical environment

This means architectural designs that include gardens, open outdoor spaces, and the skilled use of colours to reduce confusion and anxiety in people living with dementia. Try to find and support the basic needs of your patients. Some will have a low noise tolerance and others need contrasting colours to discern objects.

Individuals living with dementia often develop significant visual-spatial deficits such as shrinking peripheral vision and reduced dimension perception that can lead to disorientation and frustration.

(b) Wider operating carers' environment

The wider dementia care environment focuses on matters and priorities that mainly inform on the important developments in dementia services. These include:

- Dementia policy and strategy.
- Community support and services.
- Care standards and intervention frameworks.
- Framework on integrated support and care.

- Raising awareness and understanding of dementia.
- Community and institutional dementia care services.
- Working with new models of pathway of care.
- Dementia research and treatment.
- Stakeholders involvement.

Each of the above relates to the essential legal, policy and planning frameworks on which dementia care services are planned and delivered.

(c) The dementia homecare environment

The dementia home-based care environment has greater relevance and presents ways that may affect the quality and delivery of care. It also presents the main challenges for carers and families alike. Among these include:

- Balancing and coping with providing care with other household duties.
- Adjustment to lifestyle changes.
- Understanding the impact of dementia on other family members.
- Understanding the surroundings and likely impact on the patient's behaviour and emotions.
- Dealing with the risk of family members placing expectations on the patient, resulting in the carer experiencing inner conflict in dealing with his or her own emotions or in managing expectations of oneself or others.

- Family members may sometimes attempt to set boundaries for the patient which he or she may be unable to understand, remember or maintain – a situation that affects the emotional state of the patient and may bring about certain types of behaviour.

(d) Creation of a suitable homecare environment

The quality of life of people with dementia is mostly expressed through the experience of their environment; physical, social and the home environment. This is mainly in the nature of the communications, relationships, responses and daily interactions.

The homecare environment should ideally consist of the following key elements:

- Safety and comfort for the patient.
- Provision for their mental stimulation.
- Fostering and support for relationships with families and friends.
- Providing a calm atmosphere in the home and reassurance for the patient.
- Providing features to assist with orientation, such as memory aids for the bathroom, toilet and kitchen.
- Personalising bedrooms with brighter lights and reducing glare and shadows are simple, workable tasks that can make a big difference to residents. Provide visual and physical access to plants, special blankets or sentimental tokens, and decorate bedrooms according to individual tastes. Hang a picture of the person on the bedroom door,

or perhaps two pictures: one as an adult and one as a child or young adult.

- Providing visual prompts and symbols help people navigate their environment and helps them foster independence and autonomy. Clearly label important locations such as bathrooms, the dining room, activity areas and the refrigerator.
- Reducing risks by ensuring that service doorways and unsafe areas are camouflaged to reduce interest.
- Positioning the activity desk so that you have all residents in sight at all times. Building design and a unique personal environment are important factors that can compensate for cognitive losses. They can enhance feelings of security and promote the wellbeing of persons living with dementia.

CHAPTER 19

Creation of a Safe, Supportive and Stimulating Homecare Environment

There are key elements that go into establishing a homecare environment that is safe, supportive and stimulating in meeting the care needs of persons with dementia and in dealing with their limited abilities. An environment in which care is delivered in a compassionate setting that balances daily routines and promotes stimulation suitable for the patient's changing abilities and diminished capacities.

The essential guidelines for setting up a safe homecare environment should include the following:

- Carers and family members should try to gain an understanding of dementia, the various types and stages and how it affects the individual and impacts on the family.
- Accept the realities of dementia and the role as a carer with implications for long-term caring and to regard the caring role as an evolving process.
- Promote awareness and understanding of the patient's dementia within the family, with neighbours, friends and acquaintances.
- Homecare planning should be developed across all parts the dementia care pathway, the various stages of dementia,

and over the longer term. Care plans should also involve other health and medical conditions that may exist.

- Carers will need to realise that every dementia care situation is different and that there is no uniform or standard response of caring.
- Ongoing dementia training and skills development are an essential requirement for carers.
- Carers and families should seek to make changes or adjustments in many areas of lifestyle activities and aim to pursue other fulfilling activities.
- It is essential for carers to achieve emotional alignment with all aspects of dementia behaviours.
- Carers should seek new and fulfilling ways to stay connected with their patient, families, friends and others.
- It is important for the carer to reduce or eliminate expectations of oneself, the family and from the patient.
- Carers should aim to be emotionally comfortable and to stay stress-free by being creative.
- Carers should recognise the importance of staying connected with support groups and be able to source help whether professional, paid services or from various carers' groups. This involves the creation of a friendly space where they can interact and learn in an engaging and friendly environment.

Creating a Stable or Limiting exposure to changes in environment

It is important to avoid confusing aspects in the environment and to limit exposure to potentially dangerous situations to ensure the safety of a dementia person. The carer will need to understand that all behaviours are triggered by something, an event or some aspect of the patient's life. It might be something a person did or said that triggered behaviour, or it could be a change in the physical environment. Carers will need to identify and remove triggers that may bring about an agitated and aggressive response.

CHAPTER 20

Security and Safety Considerations for People with Dementia

The dementia persons' safety is an important priority at all times. As the disease progresses, their memory and judgment becomes impaired and they are often unable to anticipate or avoid dangerous situations. This can be an overwhelming responsibility for the carer and requires creative strategies for coping.

The carer will need to evaluate the risks and consequences of the patient's current and potential behaviour and the steps needed to ensure a degree of safety and security.

Fires are often caused when people have memory issues – not remembering they left the stove on, for example, or getting distracted while cooking. Risks of falls are also common in dementia patients and more likely in the home when coming down stairs, getting out of bed and getting into the bath. Falls generally occur due to poor balance, altered perception, and possible vision problems.

People with dementia may lose the ability to recognise objects before them or may no longer be familiar with how to use an object or where to place it, hence the degree of supervision needed has to be assessed as they become more forgetful and their judgment decreases. It is best to assess each situation individually and gradually increase the level of supervision as needed. This will help them maintain as much independence and autonomy as possible in the safest setting as can be provided. When evaluating the patient's need for supervision the behaviours to review include:

- Ability to handle emergencies when left unsupervised.
- Ability to use appliances safely.
- Ability to safely answer the phone or door when left alone.
- Tendency to wander.

Supervision practices should include such matters as:

(a) Fire safety

- Request a visit from the fire service or any professional body to carry out a home safety assessment.
- Consider disconnecting the stove and oven.
- Use of a stove guard or devise that stops electricity in the case of a fire.
- Remove or secure items that can be used to light a stove or fire.
- Actively monitor or supervise the patient's visit to the kitchen or any attempt to cook.

(b) Falls

Age-related changes can diminish balance and stability and affect depth perception, among other things. Factors that may make the person with dementia more risk to falls include:

- Chronic pain.
- Unsteady gait/balance instability.
- Hearing/sight impairment.
- Unsuitable footwear
- Medication.
- Acute diseases.
- Language/cultural differences.
- Lack of cooperation.

Responding to falls

When a person falls, a visual assessment for pain and discomfort should be done, and assistance to the individual provided as necessary. Regardless of how the fall occurred, every situation is unique and potentially serious. Therefore:

- Make the person as comfortable and reassure them, keeping them as calm as possible.
- Look for swelling and skin tears.
- If head is on the floor, it may help to place a small pillow or folded towel under the head.
- Stay with the person until help arrives.
- Even if they say they are not hurt, try to keep them on the floor until help arrives.

Preventing falls in the home

1. Ensure lap rugs do not go all the way to the floor, so the person does not trip over when they stand up.

2. Ensure the floor area is free of clutter and spills.
3. Avoid boredom among patients by giving them things to do they enjoy.
4. Provide a safe alternative for non-compliant individual.
5. Secure unstable tables and furniture.
6. Consult with occupational therapists and other professionals.
7. Exercise caution when transferring the person from sofa to dining chair or vice-versa.
8. Request a visit for a home safety assessment.
9. Remove loose carpets/rugs and clutter.
10. Install devices such as raised toilet seats, handle bars, bath chairs, non-slip mats.
11. Encourage the use of walking devices such as a walker.
12. Lock away sharp objects like knifes, razors.

(c) Reducing risks

- Ensure that service doorways and unsafe areas are camouflaged to reduce interest.

(d) Other steps

- Simple reminder phone calls for medications.
- Use of alarms on doors to prevent exiting.
- Maintain personal supervision to prevent physical injury or harm.
- Use of electronic devices to monitor and detect patient's whereabouts.

SECTION VI

Maximise Opportunity for Carers Independence, Wellbeing and Lifestyle

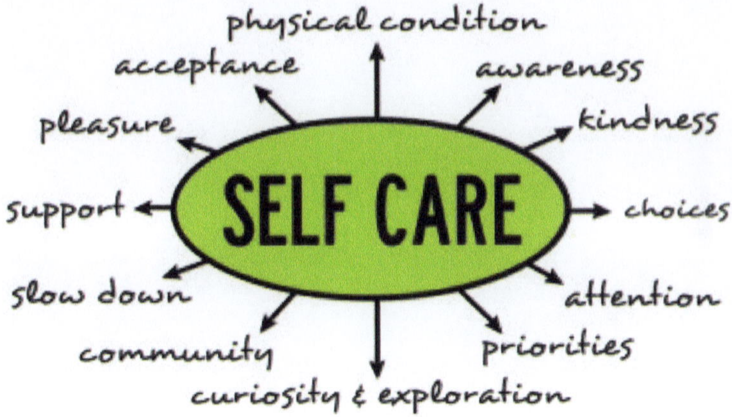

CHAPTER 21

Recognising the Needs of Carers-
Support and Resource Model

Some key facts about carers:

- Carers provide ongoing unpaid support to people who need it because of their disability, chronic illness, mental ill-health, dementia or frail age.
- Carers support people in living independent lives, to remain in their own homes and in their own communities. This care is fundamental to family life and community wellbeing.
- An unpaid carer is critical to the sustainability of the health and social services systems.
- Carers are as diverse as the rest of the community and cultural factors impact on caring. People from culturally and linguistically diverse backgrounds may have different expectations about how and who will provide care.

Design of the support and resource model for carers

Given the nature of dementia stages involved and the impact on behaviour and emotions, it would be difficult to suggest a particular model of care. The type of care and support needs of the patient, carer and family will evolve with the progression of the disease. Where there are related medical and mental health conditions, such as incontinence or confusion, these will need to be catered for in the daily care plan.

There are two parts of the care and support model to be considered for carers of dementia homecare delivery:

- Care and support model of care.
- Intervention and resource model of care.

The design and delivery of dementia care and support model should be based on a system of care and services that are anchored in:

i) The care and support needs of person with dementia.
ii) Needs, priorities and expectations of carers.
iii) Needs and concerns of families.

There are several elements that form the care and support model for carers of people with dementia. Such a model should be designed in a form that ensures carers' lives and opportunities are significantly improved, and services are effectively considered to meet their needs. Support and service plans must remain sustainable and new initiatives developed. This includes a model that is:

- Based on a diverse range of caring situations.
- Achieves national consistency and local flexibility.
- Person-centred and family-oriented.

- Determined on assessed needs and priorities of the patient.
- Ensures the delivery of safe and quality care.
- Integrated and co-ordinated with other care and diagnostic packages.
- Takes into consideration customs, practices, ethnic and other preferences.
- Empathetic and compassionate.
- Timely, accessible, responsive and supportive.
- Capable of responding to carer and family needs.

Recognising the needs of carers: intervention and resource model

The intervention and resource model for carers and families includes thirty-three dimensions of support and service needs, expectations and outcomes, with a focus on services and systems that work for carers, recognising and supporting carers in the wider community, financial wellbeing of carers, delivery and standard of care and support.

The key dimensions of support and services include:

- Person with dementia and carers assessment focusing on level and quality of care: being listened to.
- Friendly, supportive environments with access to high-quality information and activities.
- Information, advice and support provided to carers and families are useful, relevant, need-based and accessible.

- Ease of financial burden: being able to deal with the financial impact of caring, given the quality and level of care and support needed.
- Access to information and early support after diagnosis.
- Skills and knowledge for dementia care tasks, and skills training and capacity pathway of carers developed.
- Collaborative and integrated carer supports and services.
- Being aware of the growing demands facing carers.
- Referral for specific services based on needs.
- Provision of practical aids in the home.
- Carers having access to peer support groups.
- Emotional and crisis support.
- Advocacy services.
- Able to be provided with accessible and flexible respite breaks, including emergency and planned respites.
- Day care and day opportunities for people with dementia.
- Social and leisure opportunities for carers.
- Referral or signposting to other services.
- Recognition and acknowledgement of carer's role.
- Progression monitoring for persons with dementia and for carers and families.
- Provision of or access to advice and information in areas of benefits/allowances, lasting power of attorney and other legal frameworks.
- Acknowledgement, respect, recognition and rights within the community.
- Building healthier lives: attention to wellbeing and wellness.
- Understand and respect of cultural background.

- Participation and inclusion: taking part in the community and feeling included in the services on offer.
- Recognition to make choices about what carers want to do;
- Right to provide feedback and complaints about the services received.
- Finding and using services that are fair and able to access the services needed.
- Having staff who are well trained and good at their job.
- Health checks through a registered system for carers.
- Using the evidence and experience of carers to inform future policy and decision-making.
- Needs are assessed holistically with agency guided by prescribed list of services.
- Remove barriers to accessing support and services.
- Need for caring situation that requires flexibility and a personalised response.
- Assessment process should focus on the needs of informal carers and the person they care for rather than solely the diagnosis of the person being cared for.
- Outcomes planning: how persons with dementia are supported with their needs.

Care and support needs of carers during early diagnosis with dementia

The care needs provided and delivered are usually determined by assessment based on condition of the patient and includes the extent of functional disability, behavioural manifestations and memory and cognitive decline. This is coupled with the medical and mental condition that may be present at the time. The result of the assessment is used to determine what kind of assistance and care needs a person may require on a daily basis.

The care and support needs of dementia patients are based on:

- Personal care tasks or basic activities for daily living.
- Instrumental activities of daily living that require complex skills for tasks needed to successfully live independently.
- Activities that provide and support cognitive stimulation or other forms of active engagement in leisure or creative endeavours.
- Support that targets intervention or response in crisis situations.

Persons with dementia may be classed as 'independent', those who are 'dependent', and those 'who may need help' with their daily personal and other care needs.

CHAPTER 22

Building the Resilience of Carers and Families

Understanding carers' resilience

For most of the time carers are challenged by physical health problems, stress, anger, frustration, depression, social isolation and low self-esteem. These are commonly regarded as symptoms of 'compassion fatigue' or burnout.

Resilience is the way we cope with stress and adversities in life. It is the capacity to recover quickly from difficulties by learning new ways of thinking, behaving or interacting with others, thereby developing ways to cope even when life becomes challenging.

For carers for people with dementia or Alzheimer's, resilience is made up of determination, strength, flexibility, choice, support and self-compassion.

Building the resilience of carers

There are a number of ways that enable carers to build their resilience so as to best enable them in their caring role. As long as they make a commitment to take care of themselves throughout each day and week, they have the energy to avoid the daily physical exhaustion and fatigue that can diminish the ability to feel empathy and compassion for a person. Carers must focus on meeting the physical and emotional needs that result from the constant demands of caring.

At the heart of compassion fatigue is self-care. Placing their needs last can cause an imbalance between activities that nourish them and those that deplete strength. It is possible to deliver optimum care without compromising wellbeing. Being aware, recognising the signs early, and openly discussing their needs may prevent the condition going further.

It is important for carers to stay healthy and commit to self-care practices by finding calm and quiet moments in the morning, afternoon and evening where possible.

Building the resilience of carers involves the following disciplines, approaches and practices:

(i) Developing a 'sense of care', self-care is an important feature for all carers. This focuses on carers:

- Having the feeling of belonging.
- Having the feeling of inclusion.
- Forming and nurturing relationships.

(ii) Trying to understand oneself better with the focus on self-esteem, self-image, self-worth and self-respect.

(iii) Carers as humans experience various emotions in life. These emotions may be negative, producing low energy, or positive, producing high energy that makes them feel good. Carers are expected to have a range of emotions.

(iv) Striving to recharge oneself – that is, believing that looking after yourself or thinking of yourself as important. It's okay to think about you.

(v) Showing consideration and understanding when the behaviour of the person you are caring for is challenging. Try to understand what is going on with the person and how to respond. Also strive to be able to predict some of what is likely to happen in the future.

(vi) Believing that you have the ability , skills and support to take care of the things that are within your control.

(vii) Understanding our thoughts. Our automatic thought is about how we read or think of our situation, but our thoughts are not facts, they are based on our core beliefs about ourselves, others and the world we live in.

(viii) Despite the caring role, strive for a more mindful response than a reflex action.

(ix) Mindfulness, either with an instructor or online, is a self-care activity well worth trying. There are various ways to calm your mind with self-hypnosis, guided imagery, meditation, and gentle exercises.

The process of building resilience of carers also requires answers to four fundamental questions that need to be addressed:

(a) What are your core beliefs? (They generate rules for living.)

These can be:

- Negative or positive.
- They affect thoughts and behaviour.
- Extreme and inflexible.
- Affect our thoughts and behaviour.
- Produce rigid rules and demands.

(b) What are your values?

This can be answered in terms of:

- Family-oriented.
- Self-development.
- Gaining recognition for what you do.
- Gaining self-respect.

(c) What is important to you?

This tells you who you are.

(d) What are your needs?

In addition to your basic needs this can be answered in terms of:

- Social acceptance.
- Have quality time with a loved one.
- Not wanting to feel guilty.

(x) Social support groups provide opportunities for carers to remain engaged in the community and pursue their interests. They cater for senior carers and those living with disabilities. Social support groups meet regularly for various activities, usually organised according to the wishes and interests, skills and abilities of the people they are designed for. These meetings create opportunities for carers to socialise, form friendships, and strengthen function and cognitive skills. Support group activities can include conversation, meet-ups, outings, entertainment and themed celebrations, amongst many other things.

(xi) Finally, choose your response, and the attitude that you can learn to carry on. Then breathe deeply and take a step forward.

CHAPTER 23

Practising Self-care to Avoid Compassion Fatigue or Burnout

What is compassion fatigue or carer burnout?

Compassion fatigue is characterised by a profound emotional and physical exhaustion that can diminish the ability to feel empathy and compassion for whom care is delivered, thus defeating the purpose of the caregiver's role.

Caring for a person with dementia can be an intense and fulfilling experience, but it can also be demanding and stressful. Compassion fatigue is the emotional, physical and mental apathy that results from the constant demands of caring for a person and from being overly empathetic. It has been described as 'running on empty', and happens when the carer focuses on meeting the physical and emotional needs of the person cared for at the expense of his/her own needs.

Compassion fatigue is also known as burnout. Both conditions are common in caring, although it is believed that compassion fatigue is more pervasive. While compassion fatigue is easily treatable, burnout is more complicated, and sometimes a change of environment is necessary to abate the symptoms.

Carers are at a high risk of experiencing compassion fatigue or burnout, which can cause serious emotional and physical side effects. Among these are:

- Increased feelings of depression and/or anxiety.
- Anger or mood swings.
- Feelings of isolation or resentment.
- Increased blood pressure.
- Weakened immune system.
- Exhaustion (mental and physical).
- Irritability, anger, guilt.
- Insensitivity (lack of concern for the feelings of others).

Beyond those serious side effects, compassion fatigue or burnout can cause additional complications for people who work in the dementia care and support profession. For example, a person may experience:

- Decreased creativity – not good for planning meaningful activity calendars.
- Increased fatigue or exhaustion – not good for leading groups that people love.
- Decreased patience – not good for stressful trips or events.
- Disorganization – not good for documentation compliance or advanced planning.

Symptoms of compassion fatigue

The symptoms of compassion fatigue and burnout are the same:

- Exhaustion (mental and physical).
- Irritability, anger, guilt.
- Dissociation.
- Gloomy and withdrawn.
- Disillusioned with being a carer.
- Loss of purpose.
- Insensitivity (lack of concern for the feelings of others).

Managing compassion fatigue

At the heart of compassion fatigue is self-care. Placing your needs last can cause an imbalance between activities that nourish you and those that deplete your strength. Combine that with personal problems and the vulnerability compounds. Being aware, recognizing the signs early, and openly discussing your needs with peers and friends may prevent the condition going further. These are some point to consider:

- Acceptance – compassion fatigue can happen to anyone.
- Sort out personal problems.
- Assess and improve workload.
- Take regular breaks on long shifts.
- Ask others in your workplace for support.
- Peer support and proper debriefings are essential.

It is possible to deliver optimum care without compromising your wellbeing. If you are feeling 'on edge' ask yourself: On a scale of 1 to 10, how serious is this? If it is 8 or 9 over a period of days or weeks, talk to someone, share your feelings. Life-balance builds resilience, so reach out for help. Also, address your personal issues. Starting the day stressed is no way to start a day's work. Remember that self-care habits include good nutrition, sleep, daily practice of relaxation (mindfulness or yoga), and nurturing activities.

The self-care solution

Carers can avoid compassion fatigue or burnout by practicing self-care. But what is self-care?

It's anything the dementia carer does that makes him/her feel cared for. When you make time for self-care, you give yourself the rest, love, and attention you need in order to be the best carer possible. In any case, a carer needs to keep healthy and ready to take on the challenges of daily care tasks. If the carer makes his/her own self-care a priority, scheduling in time each day or week, this can:

- Lower perceived stress levels.
- Feel emotionally equipped to handle bad days.
- Be more creative and ready to try new things.
- Have the energy to smile through that next meeting with the difficult family.
- Provide encouragement to your fellow carers when they feel overwhelmed.
- Come up with solutions to problems that pop up throughout the day.

- Hug an upset person instead of feeling angry at them for challenging behaviour.
- Give better advice to family members on how to care for themselves during times of crisis.

Practising self-care whilst being a carer

Self-care can look different for everyone. You have to try new things until you find some practices that work best for you. Make sure you have plenty of self-care activities that work for you, and not just one.

The practice of taking care of oneself, as a carer, should involve the following:

(i) Eat healthily. Eating healthily will keep your immune system strong and give you

(ii) Keep fit and exercise where possible. Try to engage in at least 10 -20 minutes of exercise a day. That can be anything from taking a walk to stretching and yoga at home.

(iii) Monitoring your own physical heath. As a carer you may find yourself struggling through illness and it may become a more frequent occurrence as your body becomes run down

(iv) Acknowledge your emotions. You may feel overwhelmed by lots of emotions and these may fluctuate day by day. It is important to recognize these emotions as natural and acceptable responses

(v) Make time to relax and unwind. Making time for yourself will ensure you do not become overwhelmed by the duties of caring. Give yourself at least 5 minutes a day for you, if not more.

(vi) Talk to someone connected. As we care more and more we often isolate ourselves to the extent that we hardly ever go out and see the people we once would have met regularly.

Self-care activities

Self-care can look different for everyone. You have to try new things until you find some practices that work best for you. Make sure you have plenty of self-care activities that work for you, and not just one.

Self-care activities could include:

- Walking around the neighbourhood.
- Praying or meditating.
- Taking a yoga class, Zumba class, or other exercise class.
- Curling up with a good book.
- Trying a new recipe in the kitchen.
- Going to your medical and dental check-ups.
- Talking to a therapist.
- Repeating a favourite mantra or phrase.
- Listening to a podcast.
- Eating lunch (sitting down and not on the run).
- Drinking enough water.
- Flipping through a favourite magazine.
- Treating your face to a soothing mask, or your hair to a deep conditioning treatment.

Your self-care can include other people, like spending time with friends at your monthly book club meeting. However, you should not consider chores as self-care. For example, grocery shopping alone on a Monday evening is a chore, not self-care. Your self-care activities should also not include alcohol, as that can be an unhealthy coping mechanism.

CHAPTER 24

Optimising the Quality of Life for Carers, Families and Persons with Dementia

Carers know that their own health and wellbeing is important, but that it can be difficult finding the time, energy and resources to look after themselves. Many carers are unable to use services if there is no one to assist with those they care for. While carers appreciate the need for good health and wellbeing, it may not be easy for them to understand the need to look after their own health needs and they may often find themselves delaying or failing to follow-up on important health appointments.

Carers health and wellbeing issues

Caring for someone with dementia can cause stress, leading to depression, anxiety and poor health. This may be due to the lack of practical, financial and emotional support, or constant anxiety over the care of a loved one. Lack of sleep and physical exhaustion are also situations that significantly impact the health and wellbeing of carers and families. There are the heavy physical demands of caring too – that is, the time of the carer is mainly organised around the needs of the person they care for, and they are unable to do things that they enjoy. These things all contribute to the life of the carer being restricted and poor. The challenge is to determine how best carers can look after themselves and continue their caring role safely and for longer.

Taking care of yourself whilst being a carer

Carers should practice taking an active role in protecting their own health, wellbeing and happiness, in particular during the onset of compassion fatigue. There are six important aspects of self-care that carers can adopt in caring for themselves in order to relieve the many symptoms of fatigue and to know themselves better: Carers should endeavour to:

(i) Keep fit and take time to exercise

- It can be easy to lead a monotonous lifestyle when caring for an individual who is less mobile and finds it difficult to leave the house.
- Try to engage in at least 10-20 minutes of exercise a day. This can be anything from taking a walk round the block to stretching or yoga at home.

(ii) Eat healthily

- Eating healthily will keep your immune system strong and give you energy to care for your loved one.
- Try to have one meal a day where it is a relaxed affair. Put some music on, or the TV, and sit for 5-10 minutes without rushing around doing other tasks.

(iii) Monitor your own physical health

- As a carer you may find yourself struggling through illness, and it may become a more frequent occurrence as your body becomes run down.

- Listen to your body and if it is crying out for rest, take extra rest. Ask a friend or family member or carer for help whilst you recover.

(iv) Acknowledge your emotions

- You may feel overwhelmed by lots of emotions, and these may fluctuate day by day. It is important to recognise these emotions as natural and acceptable human responses.
- You may find it helpful to talk to someone, whether a friend or a professional. Talking about you feel is a good release of the emotions and can help you come up with strategies to cope with the emotions.

(v) Make time to unwind and relax

- Making time for yourself will ensure you do not become overwhelmed by the duties of caring. Set aside at least 5 minutes a day for you, if not more.
- Engage in relaxation techniques (lots can be found online). You could take a bath or a shower, have a cup of tea, go outside in the garden or read the newspaper.

Recognise potential warning signs of social isolation and strive for social inclusion

As we care more and more we often isolate ourselves, to the extent that we hardly ever go out and see the people we once met regularly. Staying connected to others is not only a chance for us to air how we are feeling, but a chance to stay in touch with the real world and talk about something that is not dementia and caring.

There are certain warning signs that could indicate feelings of being socially isolated. These include:

- Feelings of loneliness.
- Not having visits from friends or relatives.
- Unable to pursue hobbies or interests.
- Lack of interest in attending clubs.
- No longer socially outgoing.

Social inclusion is important for every one of us. It's great to make time to talk to someone, or have someone you know you can count on. Social inclusion defines the importance of relationships between the individual carer and others around them. By making an effort to stay connected and make friends it provides for carers the following benefits:

(i) Decreased feelings of loneliness.
(ii) Decreased depression and anxiety.
(iii) Increased feelings of connectedness.
(iv) Friendships, both intergenerational and with peers.
(v) Decreased feelings of stress.
(vi) Increased coping skills and resilience to bad days or situations.

Important steps to enhance the health and wellbeing of carers and families

The following are some of the important steps that can be considered as priorities for carers' health and wellbeing, and may be adopted by carers and families, policy makers, care professionals and service providers:

- To be offered carer assessment and monitoring that addresses carers' health, wellbeing and wellness in relation to their caring role.
- Be able to access respite breaks, including planned and emergency respite breaks.
- Better access to support and services that help with the responsibility of care.
- Be able to get support in dealing with the financial aspect of caring in relation to the quality and level of care, support and services needed.
- Better able to access specialist support, health and social care professional support at all times.
- Having practical support in the home and support in the delivery of personal care.
- Carers should find time for themselves, strive to get a social life on their own, and follow their own interests.
- Carers should be given the ability to have breaks through being able to get those they care for access to day care centres.
- Raising awareness of carers' health issues amongst service providers so they can better support carers to look after their health and wellbeing.
- Developing training and support to encourage carers to discuss their own needs with health professionals.
- Carers being able to be provided with practical aids in the home.

CHAPTER 25

Ensuring Balance in Carers' Life, Roles and Responsibilities

Carers, pay attention to your emotional health.

It can be easy for carers to put their own needs last, but it is important if you are feeling tired or stressed to look after yourself so you are still able to care for the person that needs you the most.

The emotional demands of caring for someone with a life-limiting illness can be high. As a carer it is important to look after your own emotional needs. This is important so you can continue your caring role and maintain your own emotional resilience.

If the situation seems hopeless, some people find it helpful having hope for small things. For example, you may not be able to hope for a cure, but you can hope your loved one has a good day today.

Friends and family can offer significant support, but you may find it helpful to speak with a health or social care professional, or a support worker. Often someone without an emotional connection to you or the person you care for will help you see things more clearly.

A support worker or health and social care professional can help by:

- Suggesting strategies for managing relationships.

- Giving you ideas for keeping communication channels open.
- Advising you how to balance your caring role with your own needs.

Many health or social care professionals and services offer some level of support. Start by speaking to your doctor. They may then refer you to a specialist advice and counselling service, if needed.

Carers: accepting help

Often it is reported by carers that they didn't seek help for themselves as their loved one's needs were more important. Carers also felt the health and social care team were too busy to ask for help.

Remember that you are an important part of the care team and your wellbeing is vital to being able to provide support. Don't be afraid to ask the care team for help. There are other options for assistance, too, such as trained volunteers.

Part of the care and support team's responsibility is to provide you as a carer with assistance and support, so don't be afraid to ask for help.

Carers: using respite services

Carers support and respite services can help you to take a break from your caring role. Ask your support and care service about your respite care options. You could have a volunteer stay with your loved one while you take a short break. If you need a longer break, the person you are caring for could go into respite care, so you can have some time away to properly rest and recuperate.

If you are feeling distressed, frustrated, guilty, exhausted or annoyed, it is important to know that these feelings are normal. If you find your role as a carer overwhelming, it may help to discuss your feelings with your GP or a health and social care professional or service.

More general suggestions for carers

- **Get some exercise.** Do something physical like going for a walk or stretching. Try and do an exercise you enjoy. It will help you maintain your energy.
- **Get enough sleep.** Carers often have trouble sleeping. Limit coffee and alcohol, especially in the latter part of the day. Try relaxing with a warm bath or herbal tea or soothing music before bedtime. If you can't fall asleep after 20 minutes, get up and do something else then try again. Try a brief rest in the daytime if your night's sleep is disturbed. If you find sleeping difficult on a regular basis, see your doctor.
- **Maintain a healthy diet.** Sometimes this can be hard, especially if your appetite is not so good. But you need your strength, so eat a balanced diet and remember to 'treat' yourself sometimes with food you enjoy.
- **Do something for yourself every day.** List 10 things you enjoy that would give you a short break and renew your energy. Do one of these each day.
- **Be social.** Try to maintain social contact with friends, and keep up your usual activities as much as possible.

- **Practice your own spirituality or religion.** Whether it is meditation, yoga, prayer or discussion with a pastoral worker, maintaining religious or spiritual practice will help you look after yourself.

CHAPTER 26

Leisure and Lifestyle Programme for Carers and Families

As a carer or family member the main point of reference will be the assessment of your social and human needs, which include leisure and recreation. Carers and families may also need to consider their social needs, emotional needs and physical and spiritual needs. This should focus on:

- What you like.
- What makes you happy.
- What sort of activities would make you feel included.
- What activities could potentially improve their self-esteem.

Leisure defines activities an individual may engage in during his/her free time.

Recreation is any pursuit engaged in during leisure time that is organised for social purposes.

Lifestyle is the way in which a person chooses to live his/her life.

Activities in the leisure and lifestyle programme should ideally:

- Be meaningful, entertaining and inspiring.
- Compensate for lost abilities.
- Increase life satisfaction.
- Help maintain current skills.
- Be culturally sensitive.

For carers and families the key to planning effective activities is to remember that every activity you do has the potential to be meaningful. Your attitude and engagement with others in a caring situation can make it so. A good leisure and lifestyle programme should include:

- Physical exercise.
- Sensory experiences.
- Emotional and spiritual outlets.

Common barriers to activities carers may need to overcome

Being motivated to participate in activities can be challenging and common experience. To be motivated or encourage participation it is important that you identify any barriers – whether perceived or real – that might be preventing you from getting involved.

Below are some common barriers. Most of them can be overcome with the right motivators:

(i)

(ii) Feeling of inadequacy (too old or sick).

(iii)Fear of not being able to keep up with others.

(iv)Feeling pain and/or depression.

(v) Don't like to mix with others.

(vi) Lack of awareness of the benefits of activities.

(vii) Fear of making a fool of oneself.
(viii) Language barrier.
(ix) Poor health(endurance)..
(x) Skills (range of motion)
(xi) Money (to go on community outings).

Some tips to encourage or get motivated to participate in activities

- Pair up with a friend or another who attends activities regularly and invite them to attend the next session.
- If you are in pain or depressed, inform and seek the advice of healthcare professionals.
- Try to find like-minded peers, or others with a similar personality and demeanour.
- Ask a physiotherapist to assist you in explaining the benefits of movement through exercises, dancing and walking.
- Try not to be hurried in your activity routine. What you cannot do today can be done tomorrow. Try activities several times until you build up confidence.
- Try to engage a family member to attend a couple of sessions. Alternatively, seek a volunteer fluent in the language to accompany you and assist with activities.

Supporting lifestyle changes

Many carers and family members leave behind a lifestyle they dearly wish to maintain when they enter a care environment. This in turn helps to increase unmet needs.

When planning lifestyle choices to adopt, a person needs to consider habits, attitudes, preferences, tastes, moral standards, history, culture and spiritual beliefs.

Activities worth including in leisure and recreation programme

There are both group activities for group leisure therapy available, and individual activities to meet the needs of carers and family members.

Proven group activities

These include chair exercises, balloon games, hoy, quizzes, cooking, craft, painting, dominoes, coach trips, sing-alongs, happy hour, concerts, reminiscing sessions, skittles, carpet bowls, BBQs, videos, church services.

Individual activities

These include beauty therapy, walking, grooming, puzzles, listening to music, special attention, letter writing, conversation, one-on-one visits, massage.

CHAPTER 27

Helping Dementia Carers Find a Sense of Purpose to their Lives

Carers for people with dementia and those whose caring role has ended often find it difficult to adjust to life after caring, or to understand what future life holds for them. Some may be unable to find meaning to their lives having lost their sense of purpose. There are also feelings of social isolation due to the lack of contact with family, friends and the community, also of loneliness – a feeling or a perception of being alone in the world, even when people are around. Carers who are no longer active may also engender feelings of exhaustion, both physical and emotional, and decreased creativity which means they are unable to take on the challenges of daily living.

With the loss of a sense of purpose, life often becomes aimless, dull and meaningless. There is also the potential for drifting into depression.

Adjusting to lifestyle changes

Becoming a family carer for a person with dementia often means leaving behind a lifestyle that one may wish to maintain, along with encountering a lot of unmet needs. For some individuals there is the feeling of anger that their life has been taken away from them. Being a carer at the end of their caring role represents a significant transitional point in life.

To be able to adjust and plan for lifestyle changes a person would need to consider habits, taste, culture, moral standards, spiritual needs and other factors. One must also be able to identify his/her strengths, needs and preferences. This will provide carers with understanding and selection regarding their own health and lifestyle choices.

For carers and ex-carers it means seeking opportunities for relaxation, recreation, community trips, socialisation and other aspects of daily life. This involves creative pursuits of activities that will enhance physical, emotional, mental, spiritual and social life, as well as an opportunity for reconnecting with family and friends.

Finding a sense of purpose

For carers and ex-carers alike life after caring may sometimes result in:

i. Finding a reason to get out of bed in the morning.
ii. Forming creative ways to find a 'sense of purpose'.
iii. Finding ways to motivate oneself.
iv. Finding creative ways of pursuit of interests, such as to doing things one enjoys.
v. Ensuring carers remain engaged in the community or pursue their interests.
vi. Efforts to reconnect with family and friends.

A sense of purpose boosts self-esteem and self-worth, generates positivity, and makes a person feels happier.

Bringing purpose to carers' lives

Engaging carers in all of the above can be challenging both in the immediate, short and medium term. Lack of engagement and interest is a common problem, and is especially the case when the end of their homecare role may be the result of:

- The end of life of the person being cared for.
- When caring for the person with dementia can no longer be delivered at home due to progression of the condition and requires the need for institutional care.

At the end of their homecare and supporting role carers should be encouraged to find a new sense of purpose to their lives. This requires them to identify those barriers – whether perceived or real – that might be preventing them from getting involved, bearing in mind that most family carers are seniors, with many living with complex health issues and disabilities.

Some of the common barriers that carers may need to overcome include:

i) Pain and or depression.
ii) Feeling of inadequacy (being too old).
iii) Fear of being out of place and not being able to keep up with others.
iv) Lack of awareness of what services are available for carers.
v) Finding it difficult to mix with others (being a loner or introvert).
vi) Finding it difficult for those who are not outgoing.
vii) Lack of social network.
viii) Health factors.
ix) Financial hardship.

Creative activities to help carers and ex-carers find their sense of purpose

This is aimed at improving the quality of life of carers, enhancing carers' health and wellbeing, improving self-esteem, and achieving a purposeful and fulfilling life. These should include the pursuit of activities with the following outcomes:

- Provide social interaction and to promote friendship.
- Relieve stress and provide mental and other stimulation.
- Support individual carers' interests.
- Meet and maintain carers' spiritual needs.
- Adjusting to lifestyle changes.
- Produce energy and promote relaxation.
- Increase positivity.
- Nourishes the soul, spirit and body.

Carers would be encouraged to look at a broad selection of appropriate activities to meet their individual needs and interests. Some the creative ways to help carers find their sense of purpose include:

- Community social outings.
- Relaxation classes.
- Beauty therapy (face and hand massage and nail care).
- Exercise classes with music.
- Spiritual support.
- Musical movies evenings.
- Gardening.

- Starting, or returning to, paid employment or volunteering opportunities.
- Gaining new skills or interests from your caring role that you want to pursue.

CHAPTER 28

Managing Expectations and Outcomes for Carers and Families

There are group activities for group leisure therapy and individual activities to meet the needs of carers and family members.

Proven group activities include: chair exercises, balloon games, hoy, quizzes, cooking, craft, painting, dominoes, coach trips, sing-alongs, happy hour, concerts, reminiscing sessions, skittles, carpet bowls, BBQs, videos, church services.

Individual activities include: beauty therapy, walking, grooming, puzzles, listening to music, special attention, letter writing, conversation, one-on-one visits, massage.

Support and service priorities and outcomes for carers

From the dementia carers' standpoint there are a number of priorities and outcomes that are central to the planning and sustainable delivery of care and support for the person with dementia. The outcomes will be achieved through the following:

(i) Ensure and maintain the safety, comfort and dignity of the person they care for.

(ii) Maintain or improve the functions and independence of the patient through engaging him/her in daily activities as much as possible.

i) Enhance the person with dementia and the families' quality of life through social activities and programmes.

ii) Enable the person with dementia to develop skills that support daily living activities.

iii) Introduce new experiences and coping skills to increase confidence, maintain health and reduce social isolation.

Measurement of outcomes

Carers should ensure that the measurement of support and service outcomes are based on the following:

i) Outcome measurement to be designed within the carer's needs (identification process along with a service quality framework).
ii) The relevance of the service provided to carers' circumstances.
iii) Service that is integrated, including the degree of cooperation and inter-service referrals.
iv) Measure of access. For example, carers accessing service through specific channels.
v) Measure of satisfaction. For example, features of the service.
vi) Achievement of specific outcomes, such as number of carers returning to work.

Support and service outcomes for carers and families

Outcomes for carers and families caring for one with dementia may be planned using three broad approaches, namely:

(a) Carers' health and wellbeing outcomes.
(b) Support and sustainability outcomes.
(c) General outcomes for carers.

(a) Carers' health and wellbeing outcomes

- Carers are supported to enjoy optimum health and social wellbeing and to participate in social and community life.
- Carers are better able to access respite support and to engage in activities that are beneficial to them.

(b) Support and sustainability outcomes

- Carers are enabled to access information for each step of their caring journey, from the start of caring to when caring ends. The nature of information should involve: (a) Guide for carers; (b) carers' learning; (c) respite and wellbeing; (d) relationships advice; (e) rebuilding your life.
- Carers are better supported to build their capacity to be able to self-identify their needs, plan their support in advance, and to build their resilience.
- Carers are better able to access services through a channel of their choice. For example, online, face to face, or via telephone.

- Support and services are provided in different ways. Single entry points for service and support are not a desired experience for carers, e.g. carers in crisis may need immediate support

(c) General outcomes for carers

- Carers are considered as partners with other care providers, acknowledging the unique knowledge and experience.
- Carers are actively involved in the delivery of care for people they care for.
- Carers are actively involved in decisions that affect them and the people they care for.
- Carers are supported to achieve economic wellbeing and, where appropriate, should have opportunities.
- Support for carers are timely, responsive, appropriate, accessible and flexible.
- Health and social care are better integrated with the primary focus on carers and families.
- Carers are better recognised, facilitated and supported to improve their homecare experience.
- Carers expect the broader community to understand their experience.

SECTION VII

Planning for Future Dementia Care

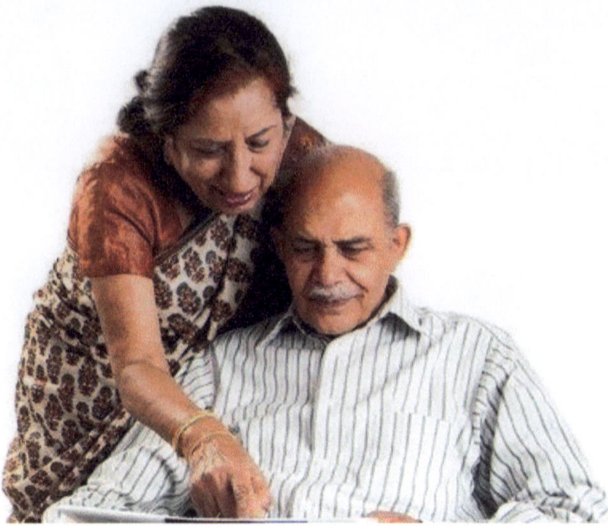

CHAPTER 29

Ways to Improve Communication with People with Dementia

People living with dementia slowly lose their language skills and their ability to express themselves freely. This has a profound impact on their quality of life and can be extremely challenging for carers, families and friends.

There are many ways that carers and families can support those with dementia to communicate more effectively. It is important to remember that how you say something is often more important than what you say. Communication is vital to our wellbeing, and patience and empathy are key ingredients. It should also be noted that every interaction is an opportunity to establish a sense of connection and improve communication and understanding in helping the person to feel safe, respected and happy.

To improve communication involving persons with dementia, carers and families need to adjust their communication style, both verbal and emotional, to make the person feels comfortable.

Communication starts with person-centred care

Finding ways to connect with the person is key. Efforts should be made get to know your loved one at a personal level to develop trust and rapport. Where possible, place them at the centre of their own care to promote independence and satisfaction. Learning about past lifestyle choices helps carers to devise meaningful ways to communicate that improve quality of life.

Successful engagement with the person is everyone's responsibility. Sharing information about past lifestyle choices among families and friends is essential to promoting positive patient engagement. Having life reflections posters or photos in the person's room are ways that can be shared, and conveys information that will stimulate discussion and positive engagement with all concerned.

An assessment provides the information you need to understand the person's interests so that you may endeavour to engage their mind, body, and spirit.

The initial activities assessment should cover:

- Reading level and interests.
- Music preferences (including type and volume).
- Past contact with pets.
- Interest in world events (news and politics).
- Religious practices.
- Cultural considerations.
- Interest in outdoor activities (nature, gardening).
- Hobbies.
- Learning opportunities.
- Exercise and physical activity.

The more you learn about the person's interests, the better you can connect with them and develop activity programmes that support them. A sense of connection and understanding is vital, as everyone needs to feel respected and valued for who they are.

Paying attention to our own body language

Some easy examples of non-verbal forms of communication are:

- Listening (active and passive).
- Silence.
- Touch.
- Hand gestures.
- Eye contact.
- Posture.
- Facial expressions.

Practice active listening

By actively listening, we are sending a powerful message to the speaker. Active listening is paying attention to not just the words that are being spoken, but the tone of voice, posture and gestures, and maintaining eye contact and nodding occasionally.

Squarely face the person. Use a physical posture that shows attention.

Open posture. Reflect on how much of your posture communicates sincerity and readiness.

Lean towards the person (when suitable) to demonstrate your participation and focus.

Eye contact expresses the message that you are interested in what is being said. Be aware that direct eye contact may not be acceptable in all cultures.

Try to be relaxed or natural. Showing that you are relaxed and comfortable assists with helping the person feel at ease.

Tips to help carers and families communicate with their loved ones with dementia

1. Realise Your Challenge. Your loved one will get worse with time. Communication will become more difficult. On the other hand, remember there will be good days and bad days. Be prepared.

2. Be Patient. Communicating effectively is one of the greatest challenges seniors living with dementia face. Tolerate any delays, adversity or provocation with compassion.

3. Offer Reassurance. Listen attentively and empathise with their concerns even if they are delusional, confused, hesitating or angry. Offer reassurance and support.

4. Minimise Background Noise. Noise can disturb and confuse people living with dementia. Find a quiet place to talk, away from the TV, radio, or people passing by.

5. Avoid Arguing. When talking, place yourself in front of your patient and speak in a clear and warm tone. Use simple sentences and give them ample time to respond. Do not contradict what they are saying and don't speak to them as you would to a young child.

6. Use non-verbal cues. Gestures, touch and facial expressions can assist communication. Observe non-verbal cues to indicate other messages. Perhaps there are other feelings behind the words they're saying.

7. Be Precise. Avoid pronouns such as 'they', 'he' or 'she'. Refer to people by their preferred names.

8. Keep it simple. Focus on one subject at time. People living with dementia cannot handle two or three threads of conversation. If asking questions make sure they can be answered with a simple yes or no.

9. Be sensitive. When talking about your patient in their presence, assume they can understand everything you say. Don't talk about them as if they were not there.

10. Take a break. If you feel frustrated, take a break. You are not perfect! A person living with dementia is very capable of reading your body language. If you do not mean what you say they will know. Taking a break will benefit both parties.

CHAPTER 30

What is Dementia?
Alzheimer's Disease versus Dementia

Dementia describes a group of symptoms associated with progressive decline of brain function, such as memory, understanding, language, thinking, judgement, behaviour and personality. There are many types of dementia, but the most common is Alzheimer's disease. Other types include vascular dementia, Lewy body dementia, frontotemporal dementia and Parkinson's. Others include Pick's disease, Huntington's and alcohol-related dementias. It is also possible to have more than one type of dementia; for example, Alzheimer's disease and vascular dementia, commonly referred to as mixed dementia. What all these diseases have in common is that they damage and kill brain cells so that the brain cannot work as well as it should.

Dementia has no single cause. Many known and unknown environmental and genetic risk factors can influence the age of onset.

Dementia versus Alzheimer's disease

Dementia is a group of symptoms and Alzheimer's is the most common cause of dementia categorised as a disease. A good way to separate the two is to say, 'Alzheimer's disease or other forms of dementia.'

Disorders that cause dementia

There are many conditions which cause dementia, and these are some of the most common types of dementia. It is also possible to have more than one type of dementia at the same time. The most common types are:

Alzheimer's disease

- Alzheimer's disease is a degenerative brain disorder that attacks the brain's nerve cells. It is the most common form of dementia, accounting for around 50-70% of cases of dementia.
- Alzheimer's disease is characterised by loss of memory, lapses of judgement, reduced language skills, personality changes and other behavioural changes.
- Occurring most often in the elderly population, the likelihood of developing Alzheimer's disease doubles every five years after the age of 65.

Vascular dementia

- Vascular dementia is caused by reduced blood flow to the brain, usually from a stroke or series of strokes.
- Depending on the severity, vascular dementia can occur gradually or suddenly. It is considered to be the second most common cause of dementia account for 20% of cases.
- Symptoms may include memory loss, confusion, poor concentration, mood changes, dizziness, balance problems.

Dementia with Lewy bodies

- Lewy body Dementia is caused by abnormal proteins called Lewy bodies that develop inside the nerve cells.
- This disease is similar to Alzheimer's disease and is the third most common cause of dementia, accounting for 15% of cases.
- An estimated 30% of people with Alzheimer's also have Lewy bodies.
- Symptoms may include lethargy, speech problems, hallucinations and depression.

Frontotemporal dementia

- Frontotemporal dementia is caused by damage focused in the front and side regions of the brain – the frontal and/or temporal lobes. These areas are responsible for our behaviour, emotional responses and language skills.
- Personality and behaviour changes are the first signs.

Mixed dementia

- Mixed dementia is a condition in which Alzheimer's disease and another form of dementia, most commonly vascular dementia, occur at the same time.
- Symptoms are often similar to and sometimes even indistinguishable from those of Alzheimer's disease.

Parkinson's disease

- Many people with Parkinson's disease go on to develop dementia in the later stages of the disease.
- Parkinson's disease is a Lewy bodies disorder.

- Symptoms include changes in memory, concentration and judgement.

Creutzfeldt-Jakob disease

- Creutzfeldt-Jakob disease is a rare, degenerative and rapidly fatal brain disorder.
- Caused by prion protein in the brain.
- Symptoms include loss of memory and coordination and behaviour changes.

Each of these diagnoses has its own distinct set of needs. Approaches to the way we deliver care will require adjustment based on individual assessment.

CHAPTER 31

Carers: Knowing the Early Warning Signs and Symptoms of Alzheimer's or other Dementias

Memory loss that disrupts daily life may be a symptom of Alzheimer's or other dementias. Alzheimer's is a brain disease that causes a slow decline in memory, thinking and reasoning skills. There are 10 warning signs and symptoms. If you notice any of them, don't ignore them. Schedule an appointment with your doctor.

Memory loss that disrupts daily life

One of the most common signs of Alzheimer's disease, especially in the early stage, is forgetting recently learned information. Others include forgetting important dates or events, asking for the same information over and over, and increasingly needing to rely on memory aids – reminder notes or electronic devices, for example – or family members for things they used to handle on their own.

Challenges in planning or solving problems

Some people may experience changes in their ability to develop and follow a plan or work with numbers. They may have trouble following a familiar recipe or keeping track of monthly bills. They may have difficulty concentrating and take much longer to do complete familiar tasks at home, at work or leisure.

People with Alzheimer's often find it hard to complete daily tasks. Sometimes people may have trouble driving to a familiar location, managing a budget at work or remembering the rules of a favourite game.

Confusion with time and place

People with Alzheimer's can lose track of dates, seasons and the passage of time. They may have trouble understanding something if it is not happening immediately. Sometimes they may forget where they are or how they got there.

Trouble understanding visual images or spatial relationship

For some people, having problems with vision is a sign of Alzheimer's. They may have difficulty reading, judging distance and determining colour or contrast, which may cause problems with driving.

New problems with words or speaking

People with Alzheimer's may have trouble following or joining a conversation. They may stop in the middle of a conversation and have no idea how to continue or they may repeat themselves. They may struggle with vocabulary, have problems finding the right word, or call things by the wrong name.

Misplacing things or losing the ability to retrace steps

A person with Alzheimer's disease may put things in unusual places. They may lose things and be unable to retrace their steps to find them again. Sometimes they may accuse others of stealing. This may occur more frequently over time.

Decreased or poor judgement

People with Alzheimer's may experience changes in judgment or decision-making. For example, they may use poor judgment when dealing with money, giving large amounts to telemarketers. They may pay less attention to grooming or keeping themselves clean.

Withdrawal from work or social activities

A person with Alzheimer's may start to remove themselves from hobbies, social activities, work projects or sports. They may have trouble keeping up with a favourite sports team or remembering how to complete a favourite hobby. They also may avoid being social because of the changes they're experiencing.

Changes in mood and personality

The mood and personalities of people with Alzheimer's can change. They can become confused, suspicious, depressed, fearful or anxious. They may be easily upset at home, at work, with friends or in places where they are out of their comfort zone.

CHAPTER 32

What all Carers Should Know

Every year 2 million people become carers in the United Kingdom, so the first thing to remember is that you are not alone. Becoming a carer can be bewildering, confusing and frightening. No one is super human, and all carers need some support and back-up. The following tips will enable carers to make people aware of their status as carers and get the support they need:

(i) Remember you are a carer

Recognising yourself as a carer is the very first step to getting the support you need. Many of us do not see ourselves as carers straightaway because we are surrounded by mothers and fathers, husbands, wives, partners, brothers, sisters, sons, daughters, grandchildren, grandparents, friends or even neighbours. We are simply doing what anyone would – caring unpaid for a loved one, and helping them through when they are unable to do things for themselves. The fact is that YOU are also a carer, and as such there are things that you need to know. Recognising yourself as a carer can be the gateway to getting a range of help and support.

(ii) Include your family and friends

Many carers turn to family and friends for support and to help them take a break from caring. It is very important that you do not try and cope alone as this can impact on your own health.

Speak to family and friends and make sure that they know the extent of your caring role. Many family members or friends may not realise the level of care you are providing, and they may be embarrassed or don't want you to think they are interfering. Other people may be reluctant to ask if you need help in case you get the wrong end of the stick and think they are saying that you can't cope! Sadly, some people don't know how to react to illness or disability and they find it awkward. Therefore, the onus is on YOU as the carer to make the moves.

(iii) Tell your doctor/GP

Please make sure that you tell your doctor or GP that you are a carer and ask them to write the details on your medical notes. A good GP will ensure that, as a carer, you receive regular health checks and also offer special flexibility with appointments. He or she should also be more willing to make home visits. Carers are usually busy and sometimes don't find time for their own health and therefore a good GP, who understands carers, can be a gateway to getting all kinds of help such as counselling, other medical services, and referrals to Social Services and other agencies.

(iv) Tell Social Services

Social Services (for adults and communities) are part of your local council and provide a range of services to carers and people with physical or mental disabilities. They should be one of your first contacts as it is important that they know about the person you are caring for. As a carer you are ENTITLED to a carer's assessment which looks at your needs and how you as a carer can be supported. They can provide replacement care to give you a break (respite), help with aids and adaptations to make life easier, or simply be a backup in an emergency. Don't just put up with new difficulties. Ask for information, help and advice to cope with problems.

(v) Tell people at work

As a working carer you are likely to need a range of support at different times, from freedom to make telephone calls to check on the person you care for, to arranging time off work for hospital discharges etc. Telling people at work that you are a carer is not always an easy step to take, and you might feel telling them depends on whether your employer is likely to be sympathetic and supportive. You can find out by asking colleagues, a personnel officer or even your own union representative, if you have one. There may be existing support available, which you might not be aware of, or you may find that your employer is willing to explore ways to support carers. You may also find that other colleagues are also carers and talking to them could be beneficial.

(vi) Claim your entitlements/allowances/benefits

We all know that the benefit system is extremely complex and many carers are unsure as to what they should be claiming. A lot of carers are put off claiming by means testing or filling in complicated benefit forms. But carers should always remember that the benefit system is there to help you access what you are ENTITLED to claim. There are a number of benefits available to carers, and one of the most important things is to ensure that the carers have the relevant information.

(vii) Find your nearest carers group or centre

Carers' groups and carers' centres give advice and support to carers by providing relevant information, arranging social events, and giving carers the opportunity to speak to other carers about their experiences. All the carers we speak to find these groups to be a great source of support. Talk to other people with dementia, or families and carers who are facing similar problems. Try to make life as full and enjoyable as possible. Both people with dementia and carers should try to get out and about and keep in touch with friends.

(viii) Look after yourself

It is easy to neglect yourself when you are busy caring for someone. However, as a carer it is very important that you look after yourself. At the very least you will not be much use to the person you care for if you make yourself ill through caring. Sadly, 1 in 5 carers report that their health suffers as a direct result of caring. Many of the most serious health problems carers suffer from, such as heart disease or mental breakdown, are a direct result of stress. Caring without a break, without proper sleep and without support can be extremely stressful. It is very important that you recognise this and take it seriously. Remember that a little help can go a long way so, when you can, try and take some time out to do something for yourself: read a magazine, visit a friend, watch a TV programme or go for a walk.

(ix) Think about the future

It may be hard to contemplate but there will come a time when you are no longer a carer. When caring ends it can be extremely hard. By facing the future and thinking about the life after caring, you can minimise the shock when the time comes. Many people say that when caring ends, they feel adrift, without purpose or direction.

ADDENDUM

Professionals Within the Community Health and Social Care System for Carers and Families to Know

Social service practitioner (s)
Care manager
Family doctor/GP
Psychiatrist/geriatrician
Community nurse
Community psychiatric nurse
Practice nurse
Occupational therapist
Podiatrist
Physiotherapist
Community dentist
Day care manager
Dietician/nutritionist
Optician and hearing aid specialist
Emergency services

If you need the ambulance service, fire service or police assistance in an emergency **call 999.**

Urgent medical care If you need medical help fast but it's not an emergency, **call 911.**

Useful Organisations

Department for Work and Pensions
Website: www.dwp.gov.uk

Alzheimer's Society
Website: www.alzheimers.org.uk
Helpline: 0300 222 11 22
Enquires@alzheimers.org.uk

Dementia UK
www.dementia.org
Helpline:0800 888 6678

Carers UK
www.carersuk.org.uk
Helpline: 0808 808 777

Carers Trust
www.carers.org
Info@carers.org

Age UK
www.ageuk.org.ulk
Helpline: 0800 055 6112

Rare Dementia Support
www.raredementiasupport.ory
contact@raredementiasupport.org

Court of Protection (COP)
www.courtofprotectionenquires@hmtcs.gsi.gov.uk
contact:0300 456 0300

Office of Public Guardian (OPG)
customerservices@publicguardian.gsi.gov.uk
0300 456 0300

Care Quality Commission (CQC)
enquires@cqc.org.uk
03000 616161

Carers Trust
Info@carers.org
www.carers.org
0300 772 9600

Glossary of Terms for Carers, Families, Social and Healthcare Professionals and Service Providers

Glossary of terms used by carers, families, health and social care professionals working in dementia homecare and community care settings. It is not a complete list but may be used as a reference point for newcomers to the caring role.

A glossary of terms enhances understanding and communication among care providers and promotes improved dementia care.

Access: Ability of people to reach or use health and social care services. Barriers to access can be (i) a person's locality, income or knowledge of services available, or (ii) by the acceptability or availability of existing services.

Activities of Daily Living: Activities of Daily Living (ADL) are basic activities necessary for independent living; eating, bathing, and toileting, for example.

Adult day care/day care centre: A non-residential facility that supports the health, social and daily living needs of adults in a professionally staffed group setting.

Advocacy: Means having someone who will express your views and wishes, secure your rights and represent your interests. It safeguards people who are vulnerable by speaking up for them.

Alzheimer's disease: Progressive, degenerative disease of the brain that causes dementia.

Approach to carer's support: The approach is to empower the person with dementia and their family to remain in control through the duration of the illness, thus helping to avoid crisis and delaying the need for admission to institutional care.

Assessment: This is simply a discussion between a person and a social work professional that helps to identify what help and support is needed for coping with life on a day-to-day basis and living independently at home.

Attendant care or homecare: Personal care for people with special needs in non-institutionalised settings.

Attorney: A person appointed to act on behalf of another individual.

Blood pressure (BP): The pressure exerted by the heart on the walls of the blood vessels. It is known as a ratio – 120/80, for example – where the first number (120) is the systolic pressure (the heart pressure when it pushes blood out into the arteries), and the second number (80) is the diastolic pressure (the heart's pressure when it is at rest).

Best interest decision: A decision that is made by another party for someone who is unable to make the decision for themselves. Must follow the best interest principles under the Mental Capacity Act 2005 and consider wishes, feelings and beliefs of the person for whom the decision is being made.

Carers: Carers provide unpaid care, outside a professional framework and within a personal relationship of family, sibling, partner or friend who cannot cope or manage with everyday living needs because the individual:

(a) Has a disability or dependency.
(b) Has a medical condition (including a terminal or chronic illness).
(c) Is frail and/or elderly with care needs.
(d) Has a mental illness.

(e) Has some form of cognition and memory impairment, such dementia/Alzheimer's.
(f) Suffers from drug or alcohol abuse.

They support people in living independent lives in their own homes and in their own communities

Carer's assessment: Carers are entitled to a free carer's assessment. The person you care for is entitled to a separate needs assessment. The aim is to give you a chance to tell Social Services about the things that could make looking after your loved one easier for you. It focuses on you as a carer and your needs.

The kind of help and support for carers that should be considered include:

(i) Respite care to give the carer a break.
(ii) Information on local carers' support groups.
(iii) Help with household or practical care work.
(iv) Carers' wellbeing, including health and safety issues.
(iv) Important commitments like relationships and employment.

Care assessment team: A group of people responsible for assessing a person who needs to be approved for government-funded services, including residential aged care.

Carers grant: This is a subsidy designed to assist the unpaid full-time carer of a disabled person to take a break from caring for that person. This means the full-time carer can take some time out for themselves. It involves undertaking a carer assessment.

Carer support: Provides reimbursement of some of the costs of using a support person to care and support a disabled person.

This means you can take some time out for yourself. Carer support is designed to be flexible.

Case conference: A meeting of all professionals (often including carers) involved in an individual's care.

Cognition: Mental processes including thinking, concentrating, remembering.

Commissioning: An approach to planning and purchasing services. The aim is to achieve the best possible outcomes for individuals who require care and support.

Court-appointed deputy: A person appointed by the Court of Protection who makes specific or ongoing decisions for someone who lacks mental capacity.

Cultural competence: The act of being sensitive and understanding to the cultural background and primary language of patients.

Court of Protection (CoP): A distinct superior court of record created by the Mental Capacity Act 2005, which makes decisions, declarations or appointments of deputies on financial and/or health and welfare matters for people who are unable to make decisions at that time for themselves.

Day care: A place where an individual can go to participate in activities and spend times with friends.

Day opportunities: A day opportunity refers to a service which mainly operates during the daytime and provides activities, care and support to those who access it.

Deputy or deputies: A person, or persons, appointed by the Court of Protection to make decisions on someone's behalf if they lack the mental capacity to make decisions for themselves.

Dignity: The inherent value and worth every person has the right to. Everyone has a profound desire to be treated as if they matter.

Disability benefits

- Attendance Allowance; Disability Living Allowance; Personal Independence Payment.
- Council Tax Disregards.
- Employment and Support Allowance and/or Universal Credit.

Discrimination: Treating someone differently to others because of their sex, age, race or other things.

Diversity: Recognising and respecting other cultures.

Enablement: Offering opportunities to be more independent.

Ethnicity: A group within a cultural and social system that shares ancestry, religious beliefs, language, and other traits in common.

How to get help: The needs of the person you support will have to be assessed before they can get help with equipment. Assessors can be a community nurse, occupational therapists, physiotherapists, speech language therapists, audiologists and other hearing and vision professionals. For who to contact, see the contact details in the previous section.

Integrated care: Coordinated health and social care that is planned and organised around the needs and preferences of the individual.

Interventions: Interventions are strategies to improve the quality of life

Lasting power of attorney (LPA): A legal document created by the donor which appoints one or more people (known as 'attorneys') to act on their behalf by way of best interest decision-making. In the case of a health and welfare lasting power of attorney, this gives the donor the ability to give instructions and preferences as to how they should be treated in the event of an accident or illness if they do not have mental capacity to take a specific decision. See below for further details:

- Property and finance.
- Health and welfare.
- If lacking capacity then Court of Protection application for deputyship.
- Need certain provider to confirm capacity.
- Can be overridden in in some circumstances.
- Can be drawn up by a solicitor/will-writer or self-completed

Legal guardianship: A person with legal authority and the corresponding duty to care for a person or property, or both.

Lifestyle: A way of living based on identifiable patterns of behaviour based on an individual's choice, influenced by the individual's personal characteristics, their social interactions, and socioeconomic and environmental factors.

Mental capacity: The ability to make a certain decision. A person who can make their own decisions has capacity.

Mental Incapacity: The inability to make a decision. A person with incapacity can no longer make certain decisions of their own, often because of illness or disability such as dementia, a stroke, brain injury or a learning disability. They cannot do one or more of the following:

- Understand information given to them about a particular decision.
- Retain that information long enough to be able to make the decision.
- Weigh up the information available to make the decision.
- Communicate their decision.

Needs assessment: Assessing a person's care and support needs including, where appropriate, those of their family and carer(s) It aims to:

- Look at your abilities, resources and support needs.
- Outline what disability support services are available.
- Determine the package of care and support that is needed.
- Determine their eligibility for funded support services.

Outcome: In social care, an 'outcome' refers to the goal or objective you would like to achieve.

Pathways to paid employment for carers: This is to promote flexible, supportive working arrangements for carers who want to take up paid employment. Working together with employers to increase awareness of carers' workplace needs and improve recognition of their prior learning and experience.

Person-centred care: The process of receiving support and care based on the individual needs, preferences, and priorities of the person affected.

Quality standards: A set of standards that are designed to ensure that services meet the requirements.

Respite care: The temporary institutional care of a sick, elderly or disabled person, providing relief for their usual carer. Respite is provided in a variety of settings, including residential care or in the home.

Respite services: Designed to provide short-term breaks for the carers of a disabled person, while also providing a positive, stimulating and worthwhile experience for the disabled person.

Rights to benefits: These include:

- Carers allowance.
- Carers premium.
- Carers credits.
- Carers disregard for council tax.

Rights at work

- To request flexible working.
- To have time off for emergencies.
- Protection from discrimination.

Risk behaviour: Specific forms of behaviour which are proven to be associated with increased susceptibility to a specific injury, disease or ill health.

Risk factor: An aspect of personal behaviour or lifestyle, an environmental exposure, or an inborn or inherited characteristic that is associated with an increased risk of a person developing a disease.

Safeguarding: Means protecting the person's right to live in safety free from abuse and neglect.

Service provider: This can be an organisational sub-unit, and is usually a third party or outsourced supplier, business or individual that offers service to others in exchange for payment.

Service users: Refer to those who use or are affected by the services of professionals. We use the term 'carer' as a broad phrase to refer to someone who has, or who currently, looks after or provides support to a family member, partner or friend.

Support and services: These are made up of four elements which focus on:

- Information and personal assistance.
- Support through funding rather than only services.
- Greater choice, control and flexibility.
- Stronger accountabilities.

Types of support services available:

(a) Behaviour support services are for people with a disability whose behaviour makes it difficult for them to engage in everyday routines, settings, activities and relationships.

(b) Day care services will include a range of activities depending on the provider, and what you're interested in and able to do. Activities may include:

- Daily living skills.
- Education and learning activities.
- Social activities.
- Recreation and leisure activities.

(c) Home and community support are services to help you live at home. This can help with both household management and personal care.

(d) Equipment and modifications for disabled people can support you by providing advice on the best equipment or modifications to your home and/or vehicle to suit your particular needs, providing equipment on long-term loan, and helping pay all or part of the costs of modifications to your home or vehicle.

(e) Residential care services.

(f) Other services depending on the needs of the person you support and the area where you live.

Under the Care Act 2014

- Assessment on appearance of need.
- Proportionate and appropriate.
- Have eligible unmet needs met.
- Be asked if willing to care and to set limits.

Wellbeing: Made up personal dignity (including treating an individual with respect), physical, mental and emotional health.

Wellness: A dimension of health beyond the absence of disease or infirmity, including social, emotional and spiritual aspects of health.

References

Note: This handbook outlines and analyses key issues and trends in the delivery of care, support and services for individuals with Alzheimer's and dementia. It draws on information and experiences that are:

- current and publicly available
- published extensively
- from reliable sources and evidenced based

It takes a broad perspective, including indicators that relate closely to carers and families wellbeing, physical, mental and emotional health, resilience and independence.

Birmingham and Solihull Dementia Strategy 2014 -2017

The Care Act 2014

Care Matters Green and White papers 2007

Carers UK

Carers Action Plan 2018 to 2020

Forward Carers

National Carers Strategy

Mental Capacity Act and its Code of Practice

Princess Royal Trust for Carers

Putting Prevention First

Strategy for Early Help in Birmingham 2015 to 2017

Strategic Plan: Dementia Information and Support for Carers Org.

Vision and Strategy to Modernise Adult Social Care

Safeguarding Adults (www. bsab.org)

Risk and Safeguarding Adults with Care and Support Needs (bsab)

The National Service Framework for Mental Health; Delivering Race Equality in Mental Healthcare Action Plan)

Google Scholar and Web of Knowledge

Supporting Carers along their Journey through Dementia

There are many changes and challenges that occur during each stage of the dementia condition. Caring for people with dementia has a major impact on the physical, mental and emotional health and wellbeing of carers, families and friends. They will be expected to practice ways of coping and managing the various forms of behavioural manifestation, cognitive impairment and functional disabilities in their support and caring role.

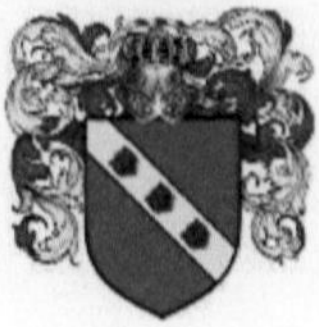

ISBN 978-1-912505-59-3

9 781912 505593 >

* 9 7 8 1 9 1 2 5 0 5 5 9 3 *
BV - #0012 - 191119 - C7 - 210/148/11 - PB - 9781912505593